Hot Pants

DO IT YOURSELF

Gynecology

HERBAL REMEDIES

Microcosm Publishing
PORTLAND, OR I CLEVELAND, OH

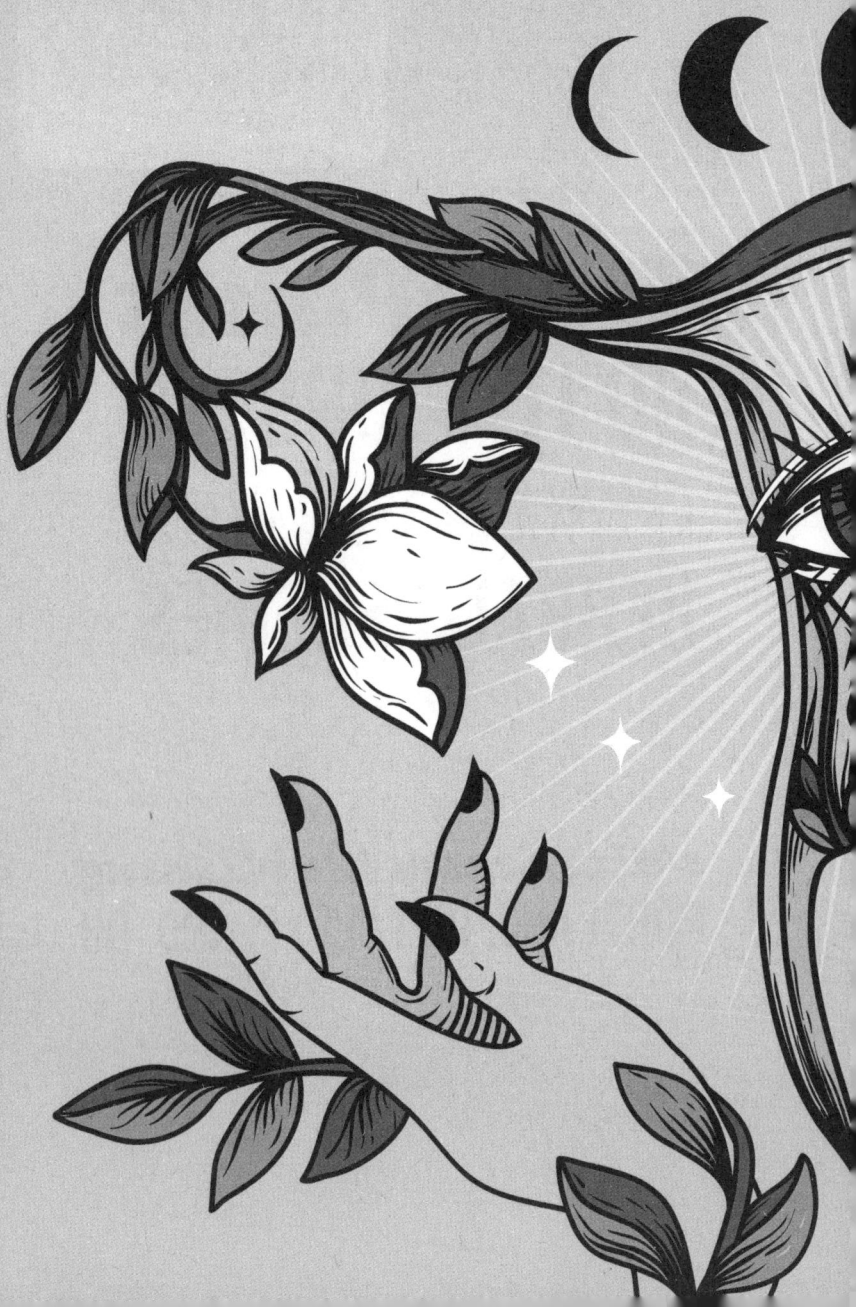

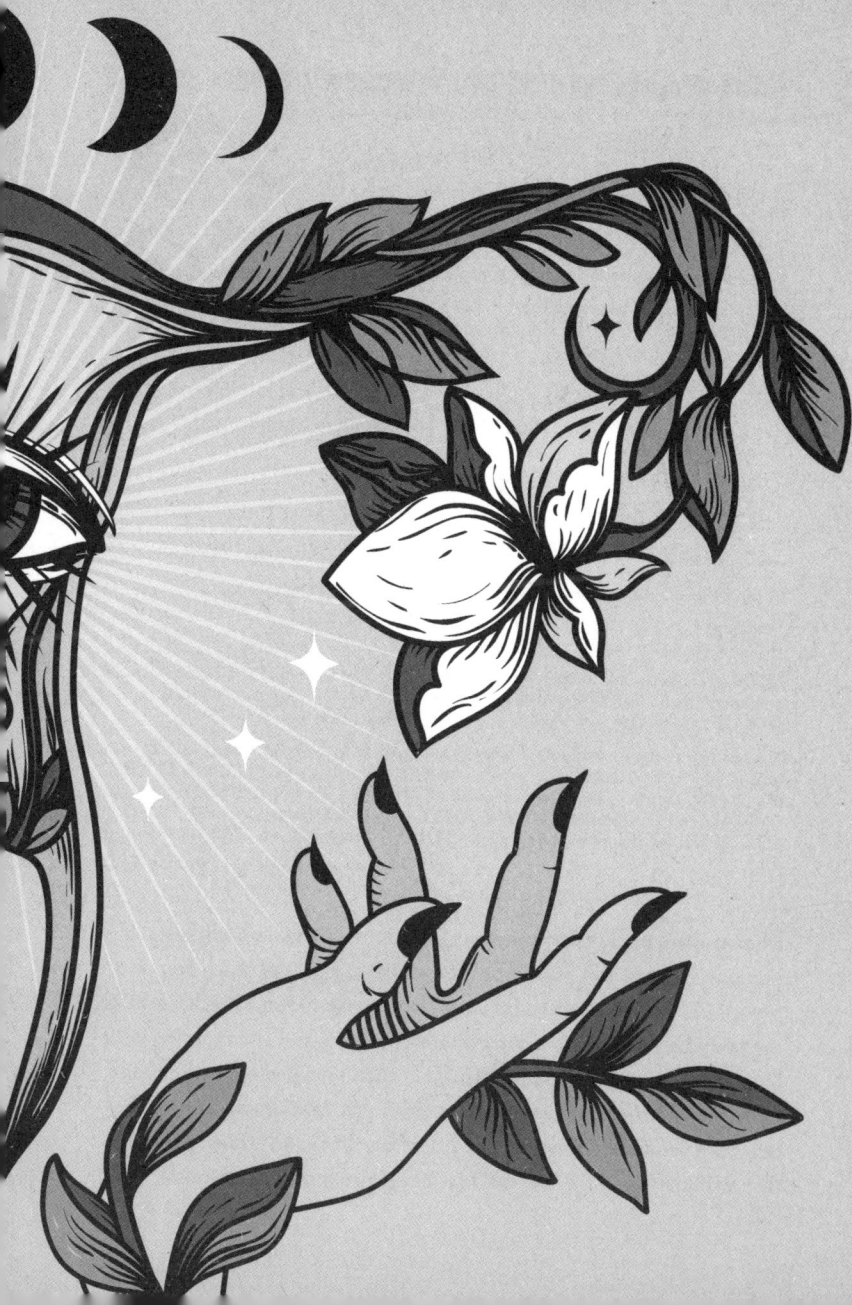

Hot Pants: DO IT YOURSELF GYNECOLOGY AND HERBAL REMEDIES

Isabelle Gauthier, Lisa Vinebaum wth Dr. JJ Pursell

ISBN 9781648416002
This is Microcosm #189
Originally published by Blood Sisters, Montreal, 1993.
This is the English adaptation of C'est toujours chaud dans les culottes des filles, by Isabelle Gauthier.
Translation by: Rachel Guay, Martine Bazar, Lisa Vinebaum, Penny Pattison, Tanya Waters, and Jennifer Petrela.

This edition was updated and first published by Microcosm Publishing, on July 14, 2015 with respect to the creation of the original publication. Third Edition, October 2025

Edited by Taylor Hurley, Chey Winters, and Sophia Cierley.
Editorial consulting and review by Dr. JJ Pursell
Illustrations by Meggyn Pomerleau, except "Anatomy: Descriptive and Surgical" by Henry Gray on pages 12 & 13, and "Fibroid of the Labium Majus" on page 57

Microcosm Publishing
2752 N. Williams Ave
Portland, OR 97227

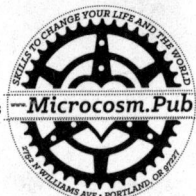

All the news that's fit to print at www.Microcosm.Pub/Newsletter.

Get more copies of this book at *www.Microcosm.Pub/HotPants*

Find more Get Your Laws Off My Uterus work at *Microcosm.Pub/ GetYourLawsOffMyUterus*

All info discussed in the following text is intended to help all people of all genders. Much of it is written in reference to women, but we intend for these woman-specfic sections to be of use to all people with vaginas and the needs that come with them.

To join the ranks of high-class stores that feature Microcosm titles, talk to your rep: In the U.S. **COMO** (Atlantic), **ABRAHAM** (Midwest), **BOB BARNETT** (Texas, Oklahoma, Louisiana), **IMPRINT** (Pacific), **TURNAROUND** (Europe), **UTP/MANDA** (Canada), **NEWSOUTH** (Australia/New Zealand), **APD** in Asia, Africa, India, South America, and other countries, or **FAIRE** in the gift trade.

EU Safety Information: microcosmpublishing.com/gpsr

Microcosm's workers and authors are paid solely from book sales. If you downloaded this book from some sketchy part of the Internet or picked up what appears to be a bootleg, please support our hardworking team by purchasing a copy directly from us and encouraging your communities to do the same. An MIT study revealed that AI inhibits humanity's critical thinking ability. Since critical thinking is one of our core values, we prohibit any use of our books to "train" generative artificial "intelligence" (AI) technologies, because seriously, WTF

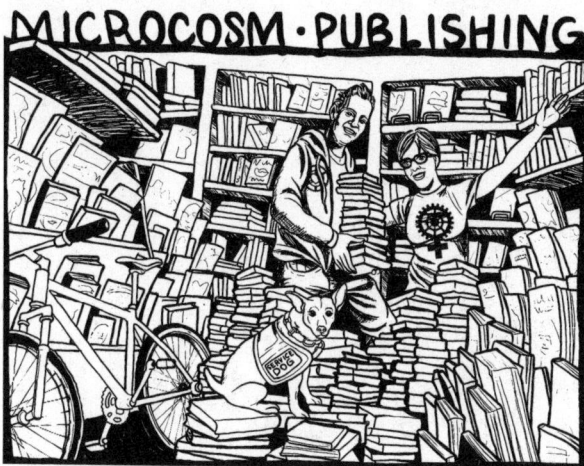

MICROCOSM PUBLISHING is Portland's most diversified publishing house and distributor, with a focus on the colorful, authentic, and empowering. Our books and zines have put your power in your hands since 1996, equipping readers to make positive changes in their lives and in the world around them. Microcosm emphasizes skill-building, showing hidden histories, and fostering creativity through challenging conventional publishing wisdom with books and bookettes about DIY skills, food, bicycling, gender, self-care, and social justice. What was once a distro and record label started by Joe Biel in a drafty bedroom was determined to be *Publishers Weekly*'s fastest-growing publisher of 2022 and #3 in 2023 and 2024, and is now among the oldest independent publishing houses in Portland, OR, and Cleveland, OH. We are a politically moderate, centrist publisher in a world that has inched to the right for the past 80 years.

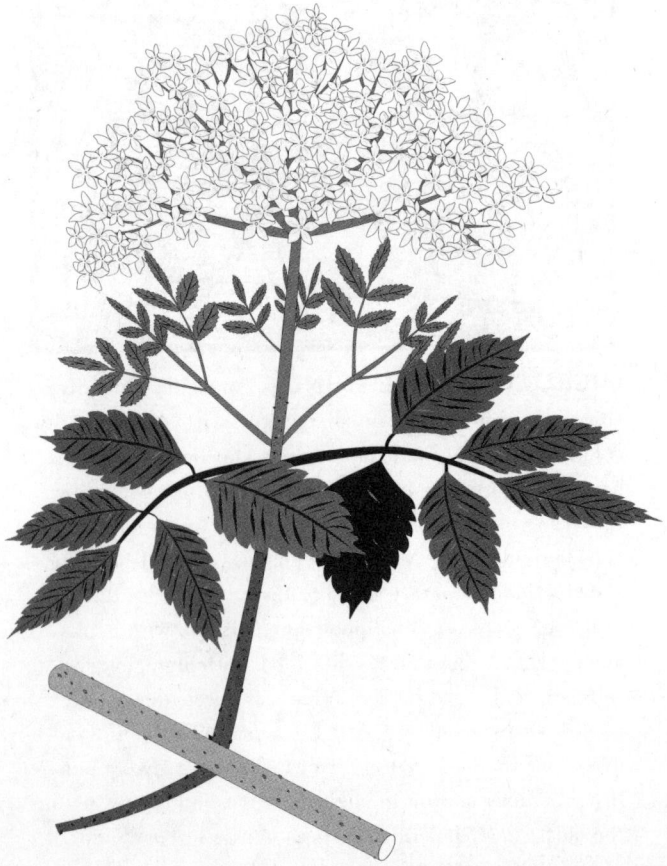

D I S C L A I M E R

TEN GOOD REASONS

IF YOU'D LIKE TO KNOW AS MUCH ABOUT YOUR CUNT AS YOUR DOCTOR DOES

IF THE PILL IS GIVING YOU THE BLUES

IF THE CONDOM BUSTS

IF ANTIBIOTICS GIVE YOU A YEAST INFECTION

IF YOU BLEED BUCKETS

...AND FOR MANY OTHER REASONS...

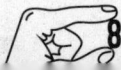

8

TO KEEP THIS BOOK ON HAND AND TO SHARE IT →

→ IF YOU BREAK OUT INTO A COLD SWEAT EVERY TIME YOUR PERIOD'S LATE

→ IF YOUR FRIEND'S GOT CRAMPS

→ IF YOU CATCH THE CLAP

IF YOUR YEASTY ITCH MAKES YOU WANT TO GRAB THE STEEL WOOL

→ IF STIs ARE SQUATTING YOUR CROTCH

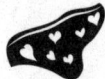

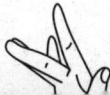

TABLE OF CONTENTS

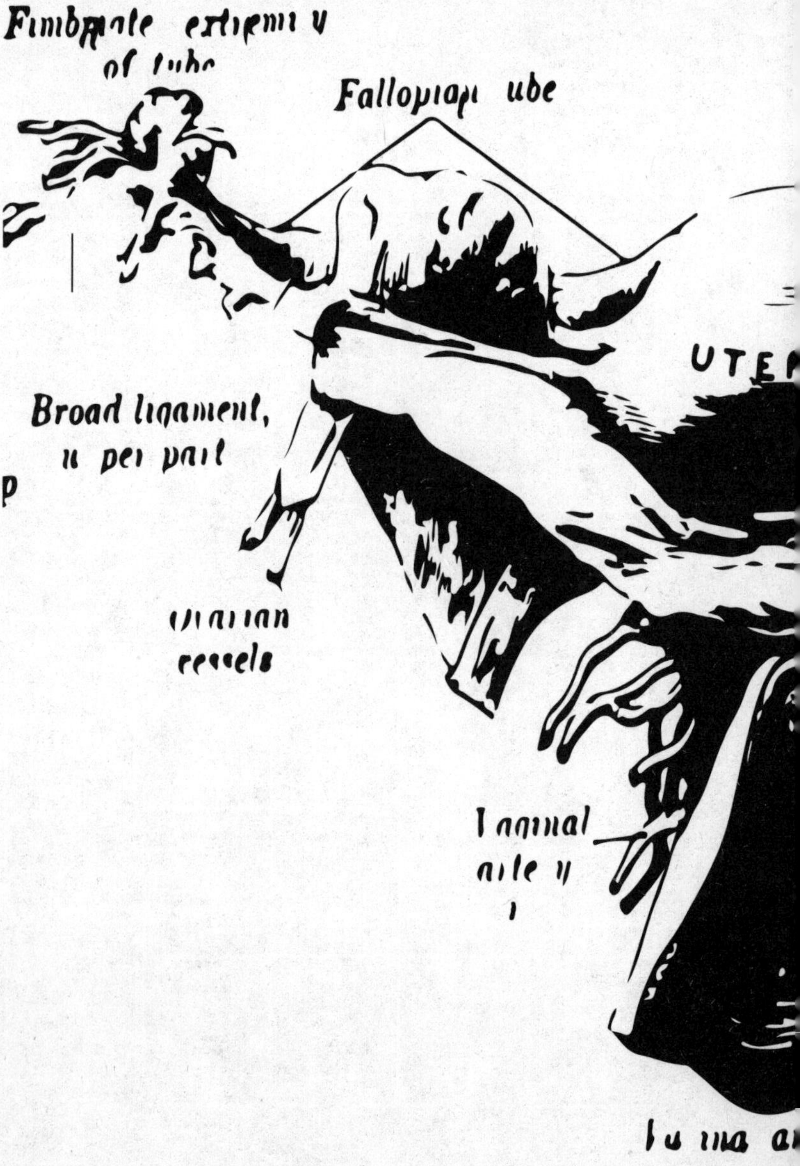

Fimbriate extremity
of tube

Fallopian tube

UTE

Broad ligament,
u per part

p

ovarian
vessels

I ngvinal
nfe y

lu ina a

12

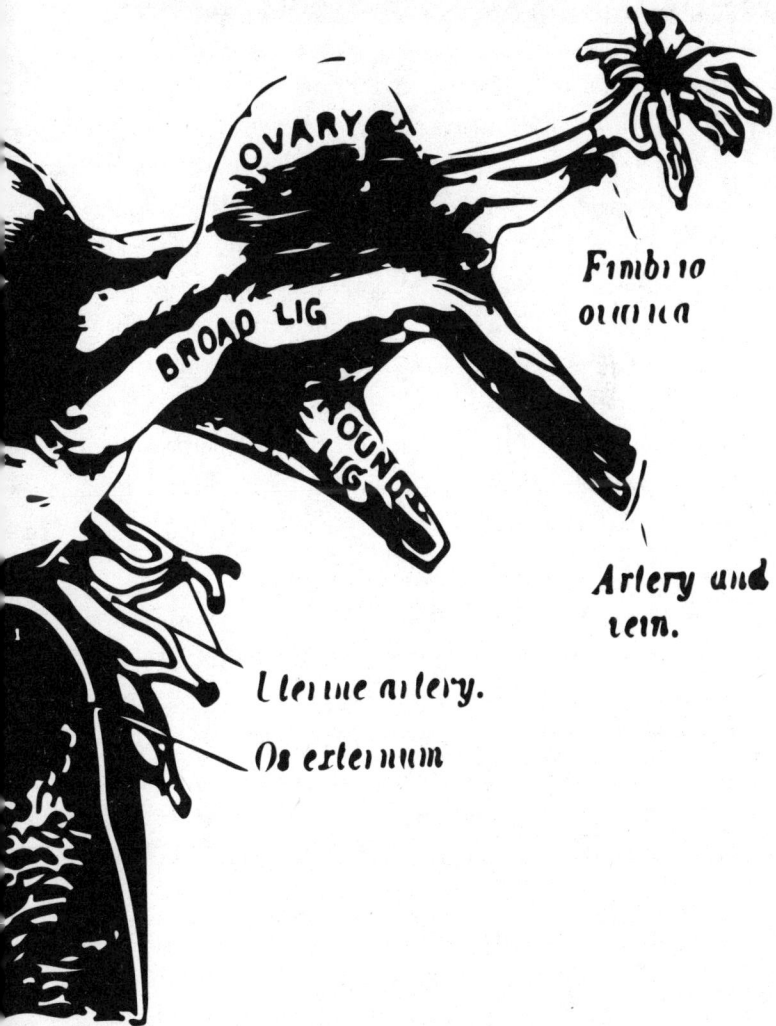

OVARY

BROAD LIG

ROUND LIG

Fimbrio ominia

Artery and vein.

Uterine artery.

Os externum

ur uutb.

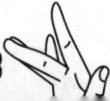

FEMINIST, HEAL THYSELF

I was lucky to grow up in the wake of the feminist health movement of the seventies, which bypassed the "experts" anointed by the patriarchy in order to put healing tools right in the hands of women themselves. In the early 1980s, long before I became a feminist writer, I was a repressed tween growing up in Fargo, North Dakota. When it came to my body or what puberty had in store, I gleaned more from reading Judy Blume books—*Are You There God? It's Me, Margaret; Deenie;* and *Then Again, Maybe I Won't*—than in all my embarrassing health classes combined. Later on—in high school, college, and my twenties—books came to the rescue more often than my annual trip to the gynecologist.

There is nothing like a book (or booklet) that you can hold in your very own hands and consult as needed to quell any suspicions that you are a perverted mutant. This is why I believe in easily passed-on owners' manuals for the reproductive system like *Hot Pants: Do It Yourself Gynecology and Herbal Remedies.* In the tradition of feminist bibles like *Our Bodies, Ourselves, Hot Pants* is a DIY pamphlet created by a group of lay-women who sought to give each other the kind of help that was not forthcoming from careless and condescending medical professionals. Originally published in 1993 by the Montreal collective BloodSisters, *Hot Pants* draws from ancient wells of wisdom and combines no-

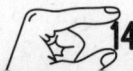

nonsense sexual health information with the basics of herbal therapy, bypassing big Pharma *and* patriarchy.

I moved to New York to work at *Ms.* in 1993, the year *Hot Pants* was born, and met many of the "health feminists"[1] cited herein—trailblazers like Barbara Seaman, Susie Bright, Barbara Ehrenreich, and Susun Weed. While I don't want to overstate the menace of traditional medicine,[2] the opening lines of *Hot Pants* are unequivocally true: "Patriarchy sucks. It has robbed us of our autonomy and much of our history," and women must "be in control of our own bodies." This harmonizes with another feminist classic, *Witches, Midwives and Nurses* (Barbara Ehrenreich and Deirdre English, 1973), which asserts that medicine is women's "birthright," as we are the "unlicensed doctors, anatomists, abortionists, nurses, therapists, and pharmacists of western history."

In this handy handbook, you'll find herbal recipes for everything from menstrual cramp remedies to aphrodisiacs, as well as concise descriptions of many STIs, a helpful glossary, and great suggestions for further feminist reading. Some of the advice should be met with a healthy dose of skepticism—you will not find me putting raw garlic or a sea sponge in my vagina—but the reassurance that I can get to know what my vagina looks like in its healthy state is pure empowerment. Their section on emmenagogues reminded

---

1 This was the term my mentor Barbara Seaman, the author of *The Doctor's Case Against the Pill,* used for her cohort of activist-healers who transformed the culture into which I was born.

2 My dad is a doctor, and, to this day, he is my go-to for all things medical and emotional.

me that the various forms of menstrual extraction[3] are crucial knowledge, especially now, with *Roe* overturned and our legal ownership of our bodies an actual thing of the past. It's powerful to know what your labia look like and how their appearance changes throughout your cycle and your life. And if you've never seen your cervix, DIY gynecology is here to say all you need is a mirror, a $2 plastic speculum, a mini-flashlight, and *voila*! This is a manifesto that embraces knowledge, feminist history, and the total ordinariness of even your most shameful secret or fear. As the authors note in their section on sex: "It's normal to change your partners, mind, and methods. It's normal to abort. It's normal to freak out! . . . It can seem bleak at times, but keep in mind that lovers come and go. Your body is yours for the long haul."

—Jennifer Baumgardner

of money, but lasts almost

strual
e (PMS)

ood changes, irritability, cramps,
reasts, headaches, zits, water
lack of energy, herpes outbreaks,
ive malfunctions, flu-like

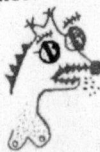

---

3 Here I'm referring to Lorraine Rothman and Carol Downer's development of the Del-Em (or Dirty Little Machine, as they called it), a device for DIY early abortion, newly relevant for today's America!

Patriarchy sucks. It's robbed us of our autonomy and much of our history. We believe it's integral for women to be aware and in control of their own bodies. The recipes we present here have been known and practiced for centuries, passed down from mother to daughter, and have survived the censorship of the witch hunts. Our intent is simple and practical: to help break away from the medical establishment's tentacular grip on our bodies and our approaches to health and healing.

From **anatomy** to **self-healing** using herbs and massage, it is filled with easy recipes and remedies to conquer **yeast infections, sexually transmitted infections (STIs), hormonal imbalances, and late periods**, among other things. A whole array of medicinal plants and nutritional information is provided to arm us against abusive and negligent medical practices. A section on aphrodisiac plants has been added for your fancy.

Because the world of women's health is vast and multi-faceted, we had to prioritize the selection of material. We decided to focus on sexually transmitted diseases, unwanted pregnancies, and more specific gynecological problems as there is a lack of alternative literature on these subjects. Other aspects of women's health (menopause, fertility, pregnancy, psychological aspects, etc...), while extremely important, are too exhaustive for us to cover here.

Staying healthy depends on good nutrition and lifestyle, even in matters such as STIs, poverty, abuse and

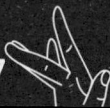

living in a crazed society make us easy targets for all kinds of unwanted invaders—including the medical establishment.

Hot Pants is an English adaptation of *C'est toujours chaud dans les culottes des filles*. The original translation, *Hot Pantz*, was a zine that has been photocopied and sold, traded, and given away for over 20 years. We found the information in it invaluable, but the repeated copying made it difficult to decipher, and some of it was out of date and incomplete. With a team of researchers and professional herbal doctors, we worked to update, revise, and clarify *Hot Pants* for modern times, while staying true to the authors' original intentions and tone. In particular, we have removed instructions for douching, which is now considered to be harmful, and included more information on topics like the dosages and side effects of various herbs.

This book is an introduction to basic herbal therapy; it's a manner of getting to know different medicinal plants and their properties, and figuring out which ones work best for each of us. Many of the treatments outlined in this book will not be enough to eliminate certain chronic conditions. If you find yourself in this situation, you may want to opt for more advanced herbal approaches. Consult books written by other witches and healers who escaped the stake. Ask a naturopathic physician, or perhaps take a closer look at homeopathy, acupuncture, etc, all of which are valuable methods of healing, especially when used as long-term treatments.

While these treatments are specifically recommended for women, many of them can also be

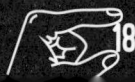

applied to men. We also would like to recommend using either organic or homegrown herbs and plants (picking wild herbs can be okay, just be mindful of their growing environment) to avoid chemicals and pesticides. We also would like to warn against douching; douching has been linked to pelvic inflammatory disease, bacterial vaginosis and infections, and an increased risk of ectopic pregnancy, among other things. While some still hold that douching with herbs is harmless, it is best to consult an herbalist to ensure the treatment is appropriate.

The last sections *"How to Prepare and Use Herbs"* and *"Herbal Properties and Dosages,"* contain explanations, methods of preparation (**infusions, decoctions, tinctures**...) and above all, the characteristics and ways of using the herbs mentioned in this book. While it may be tempting to skip ahead to the treatments suggested, it is ***extremely important*** that you read these sections. Herbs are very powerful and it's important that you understand how they work, how to prepare them, and when to avoid using certain plants.

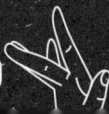

[front view of vagina]

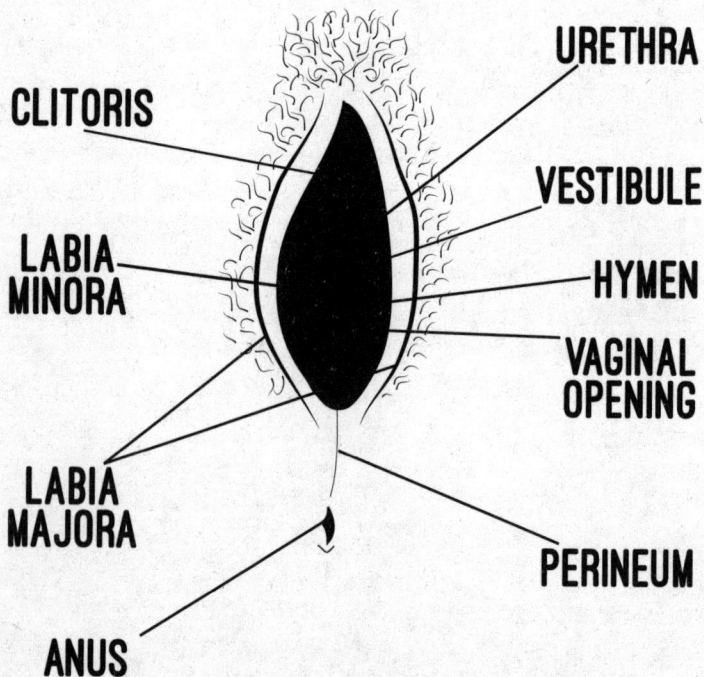

CLITORIS

LABIA
MINORA

LABIA
MAJORA

ANUS

URETHRA

VESTIBULE

HYMEN

VAGINAL
OPENING

PERINEUM

[lateral view of vagina]

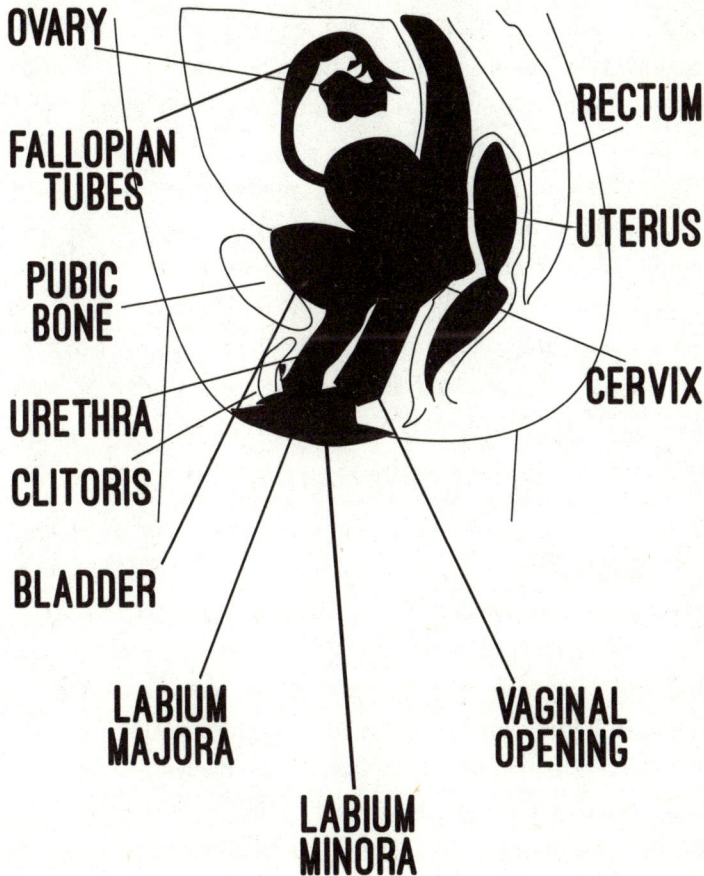

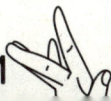

OVARY

FALLOPIAN
TUBES

PUBIC
BONE

URETHRA

CLITORIS

BLADDER

RECTUM

UTERUS

CERVIX

LABIUM
MAJORA

LABIUM
MINORA

VAGINAL
OPENING

BODY MAPPING (IN BRIEF)

The external female genital organs are the **clitoris** and the **labia**. Together they form the **vulva**. The **labia majora** (outer lips) cover the other parts of the vulva. They become thinner at their base, where they fuse with the **perineum**, the muscle between the **anus** and the **vagina**. Inside the labia majora is the **labia minora**. They are joined at the top to form a protective sheath over the clitoris. They also protect the opening to the **urethra.**

The area between the labia minora is largely occupied by a space called the **vestibule**. At birth this space is almost completely covered by the **hymen**, which varies in size, shape, and rigidity. The hymen can be torn during sporting activities, by the insertion of a tampon, during masturbation, or vaginal penetration. Some women have a piece of skin around the vestibule—this would be remnants of the hymen.

THE CLITORIS & GENITAL GLANDS

The clitoris is, essentially, an organ designed for sexual stimulation and pleasure. The clitoris and labia contain erectable tissue which swells up during sexual excitement.

Two pairs of glands are attached to the vulva; the **Skene's glands** lie just under the clitoris and secrete an alkaline liquid which reduces the vagina's natural acidity. The second and larger set of glands, the **Bartholin's glands**, are located at the opening of the vestibule and secrete fluid during stimulation. They are normally about the size of a small pea and are not very prominent. Their swelling can be caused by what is called a **Bartholin's abscess** or cyst.

THE VAGINA

The vagina is the channel which connects the vulva and the internal organs. It is seven to twelve centimeters long. Vaginal secretions are typically acidic, but during ovulation there is a slight shift from acidic to alkaline to help support sperm viability for possible conception. Vaginal secretions come from the Bartholin glands and from the **cervical canal** (which is also the source of cervical mucus). Normal discharge is odorless and watery or slightly white. Its function is to cleanse the vaginal canal, as well as coat the interior of the vagina.

THE UTERUS

The uterus is about the size and shape of a pear and is made up from two main parts: the **body** and the **cervix.** From puberty to menopause, the **endometrium** (or the uterine lining) forms every month to provide nutritive support for a fertilized egg. If the egg is not fertilized, the endometrium is expelled. This is known as menstruation. It is also believed that the uterus is the center of a woman's energy and that each month we gather up and store emotions and experiences in the womb. Menstruation is the release and cleansing of those emotions each month.

The cervix is shaped like a cylinder; it is approximately two and a half centimeters long, with a fine canal running through it, opening into the uterus up top, and to the vagina at the bottom.

All changes in the functions of the uterus (menstruation, pregnancy, menopause) are regulated by hormones controlled by

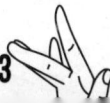

the **hypothalamus**, the **pituitary gland**, the **ovaries**, and by other substances (such as **prostaglandins**) secreted by the uterine tissue. The uterus is connected to the **fallopian tube**s, which hold the **ovum** (or egg) released every month by one of the two ovaries.

THE OVARIES

The ovaries are located in the pelvis and rest on either side of the uterus. Each ovary is held in place by strong elastic ligaments. The notched orifice of the fallopian tube is located just above the ovary, with the tube leading to the uterus. Even though they are very close to each other, the ovaries and the opening of the fallopian tube are not in direct contact; but the feathery finger-like projections of the fallopian tube have a magnetic attraction, pulling the released ovum in. The ovaries develop and release the ovum and play an essential role in our hormonal system. They are pinkish-grey, almond shaped, and about three centimeters long. A layer of cells called the **oogenic epithelium** covers the ovaries: it is from these cells that the egg is formed. Thousands of immature **ova** (eggs) gather in these pouches on the surface of the ovaries. In addition to their role of developing the ova, the ovaries produce the hormones **estrogen** and **progesterone**.

FOR MORE INFORMATION ON ANATOMY, WOMEN'S GENITAL ORGANS AND THEIR FUNCTIONS, AND ON THE ROLE AND FABRICATION OF HORMONES, CONSULT THE FOLLOWING BOOKS:

Natural Healing in Gynaecology by Rina Nissim

The Women's Answer Book by Lois Jovanovik-Peterson M.D. and Genell J. Subak-Sharpe M.S. (Ballantine Books) Down There: Sexual and Reproductive Health the Wise Woman Way by Susun S. Weed

Women's Encyclopedia of Natural Medicine: Alternative Therapies and Integrative Medicine for Total Health and Wellness by Tori Hudson and Christiane Northrup

Our Bodies, Ourselves by the Boston Women's Health Book Collective (Simon and Schuster)—especially good for info on anatomy.

ABOUT MENSTRUATION

It is surprising to realize to what extent menstruation is an individual thing—every woman menstruates, yet color, odor, temperature, needs, desires, and pain can vary tremendously from woman to woman. It is also amazing to note that women who live together or who are very close often menstruate at the same time.

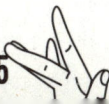

In many societies menstruation was traditionally (and in some cases still is) viewed as a very powerful time—a time for women to purify themselves and to relax. This is a far cry from how most of us experience bleeding. We're usually taught to hide any evidence of blood, pads or plugs (hence the ridiculous individually wrapped polka-dotted packaging), to be "discreet" (like, don't talk about it at all) or don't whine ("you're such a bitch when you're on the rag").

We encourage bitching, talking, and doing whatever else allows you to feel better while honoring all that is happening in your body.

A GOOD IDEA FOR REPLACING TAMPONS

Brand-name tampons and pads can be harmful to you. Plus they cost a fortune, being "luxury" items and all. Whenever possible, avoid scented products as these release a whole slew of chemicals into your girl parts (and smell gross). Tampons are bleached using dangerous chemicals which can be absorbed into the body through the vaginal walls, and not to mention **toxic shock syndrome** has been directly linked to tampon use. Plastic tampon applicators are non-biodegradable and clog sewage systems, often washing up on bays and beaches. You can avoid some of these problems by using non-bleached tampons, available at some health food stores. You can also buy 100 percent cotton pads (or even better—make your own!). They are washable and re-usable, thus avoiding unnecessary waste.

Instead of tampons you can also use natural sea sponges. Simply dampen the sponge, insert it into the vagina with your fingers, and remove it once it's saturated. If you push it up too far, there is some risk of losing it "up there." Sponges can be left inside the vagina for several hours, depending on your flow and the size of the sponge. Once the sponge is saturated, rinse it in warm or cold running water, squeeze out the excess water, and reinsert it.

This is a cheaper, eco-friendly alternative to tampons. Avoid synthetic sponges. Natural sponges are often sold as make-up removal pads, and can be found in the cosmetic section of the pharmacy or at health food stores. 'Course they aren't advertised as menstrual sponges cause that would threaten the "sanitary hygiene" industry. A sponge can last up to sixth months if you take good care of it. Discard the sponge once it begins to fall apart.

Soak your sponge overnight in a cup of water with one teaspoon of white vinegar before and/or after each period. This kills the bacteria that can cause yeast and other vaginitis. If you have a bad vaginal infection during menstruation, it's best not to reuse that sponge again. Store your sponge in a cloth or box between periods.

Menstrual cups are another great alternative to tampons and pads. These silicone cups are folded in half and gently inserted up into the vaginal canal. Once inside the fold opens up so that menstrual blood is collected inside the cup. They have a tiny tail that can be pulled when removal is desired.

PRE-MENSTRUAL SYNDROME (PMS)

These are varied: mood changes, irritability, cramps, painful or swollen breasts, headaches, zits, water retention, bloating, lack of energy, herpes outbreaks, gas and other digestive malfunctions, flu-like symptoms, back pains... Combine these symptoms with an irregular or painful cycle and you've got the most generic profile of a woman who's ready to kill. Most likely she'll be prescribed The Pill to "solve" all her problems. Medical genius at its finest...

Methods of Coping:

- Diet.
- Lower your intake of salt.
- Eat food rich in potassium: bananas, potatoes, cabbage, pears, and almonds.
- Eat a lot of seaweed: kelp (fresh or in tablet form), hijiki, dulse.
- Make foods high in vitamin B6 a regular part of your diet: green vegetables, and nutritional yeast (you can also take brewer's yeast capsules). Note that women who are prone to yeast infections should avoid baker's yeast; nutritional yeast is derived from a deactivated form of yeast and will neither reproduce nor cause infection when consumed.
- Take a lot of vitamin A, especially if you have painful breasts or suffer from cramping. Carrots, onions, garlic, turnips, spinach, lentils, apricots, lemons, and raw vegetable oils are all rich in vitamin A. Be aware,

overdose of vitamin A from supplements can cause liver damage.

- Drink lots of water!

Herbal Treatments

- Follow the treatments for hormonal imbalances on page 80.
- Take Valerian tincture found on page 116 to relax and smooth muscles in the body, including the uterus.
- Take ginger (page 105) to relieve tension and cramps
- Some books provide a detailed account of the role played by hormones in causing PMS—why we produce too much of certain hormones, and not enough of others. PMS is often caused by hormonal irregularities, and so it is helpful to read up on this subject.

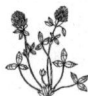 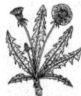 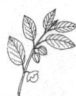

RED CLOVER   DONG QUAI   HOLY BASIL   CLARY SAGE OIL   ST. JOHN'S WORT   DANDELION   ASHWAGANDHA

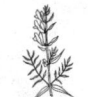 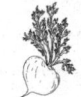 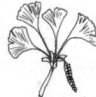

CHINESE SKULLCAP   GINGER ROOT   FENNEL SEED   BLACK COHOSH   EVENING PRIMROSE OIL   MACA   GINKGO

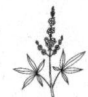 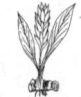 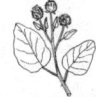

CHASTE TREE   CYPRESS OIL   CINNAMON   LEMON BALM   WILD YAM   TURMERIC   BURDOCK

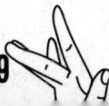

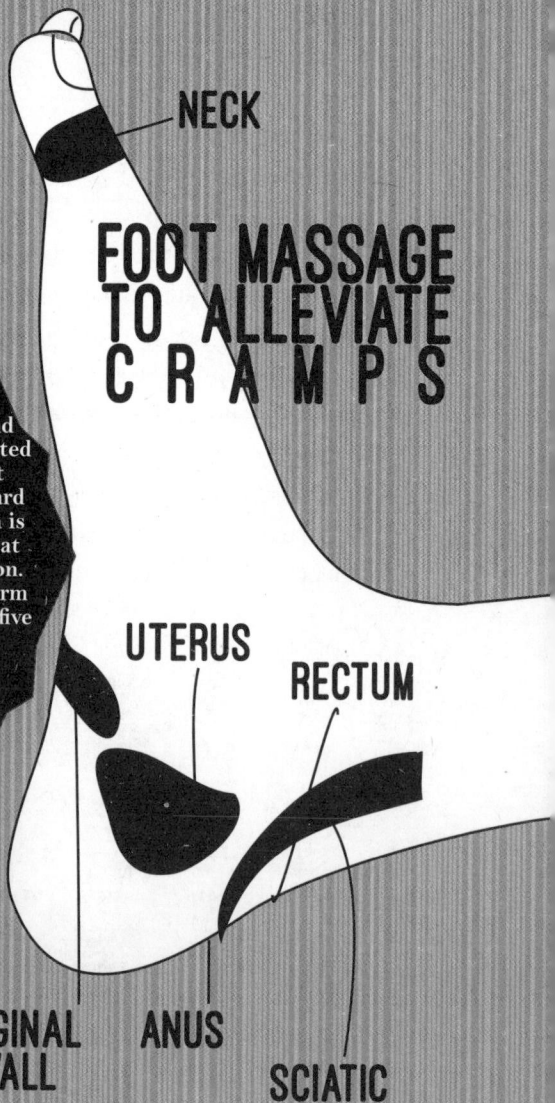

[inside of foot]

NECK

FOOT MASSAGE TO ALLEVIATE CRAMPS

Massage the uterine and ovarian reflex areas (located behind the ankles, just above the heel). Press hard where it hurts. This area is generally very sensitive at the onset of menstruation. Use your thumb to put firm pressure on the area, for five minutes on each side.

UTERUS

RECTUM

VAGINAL WALL

ANUS

SCIATIC

[outside of foot]

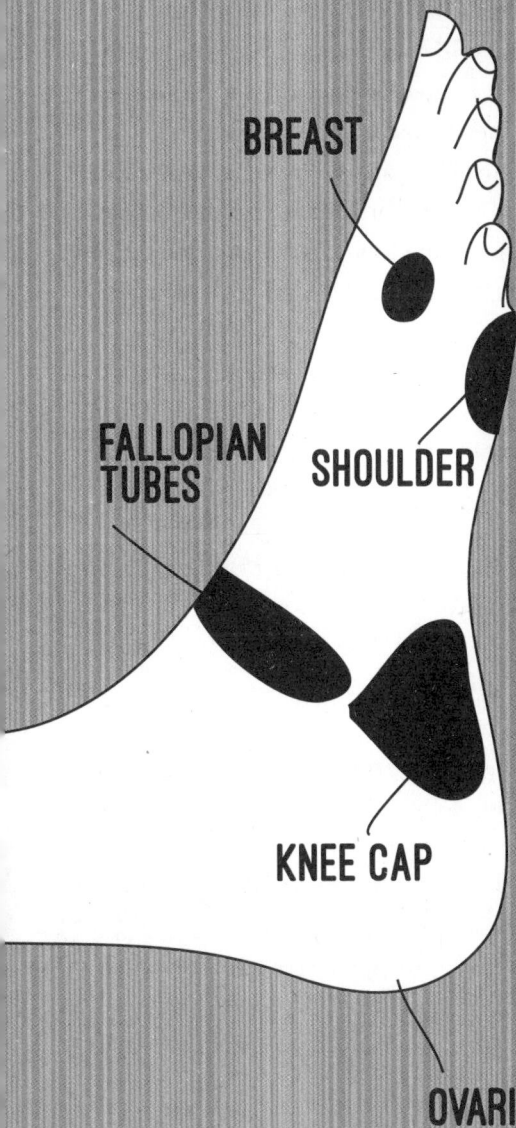

BREAST

FALLOPIAN
TUBES

SHOULDER

Alternate massaging
each foot as needed.
This massage yields
astonishing results,
especially if it's done
by someone else.

KNEE CAP

OVARIES

AMENORRHEA OR ABSENCE OF MENSES

This may be due to several factors. Normal absence of menstruation (missing a period, or several) is caused by pregnancy, lactation, or menopause.

Amenorrhea can also be caused by very poor diet, excessive exercising, losing large amounts of weight, fatigue, stress, hormonal imbalance, going off The Pill, anemia or by metabolic problems: diabetes, liver disease, or inconsistencies in thyroid levels. Try to eat well.

To Bring on Menstruation:

- A spring of parsley inserted as far as possible into the vagina can bring on menstruation by causing uterine contractions. Insert it before going to sleep, and remove it the following morning. **Do this for three to four days.** Accompany this with parsley infusions found on page 110. Again, we recommend using organic or homegrown parsley for this treatment.
- Take a sage infusion (page 113) or tincture (page 89).
- Drink motherwort (page 109) infusions (infusion found on page 110) for **four to five days. Do not exceed six days**; you should get your period in the following days.
- Massage the reflex zones for the uterus and ovaries **two to three times a day** (page 30)
- Tansy infusion or tincture (found on page 114) can help regulate amenorrhea. Note that tansy can cause heavy bleeding in women who normally have a heavy flow.

- Drink teas with herbs such as vitex, dong quai, peppermint, chamomile (page 101), and red raspberry (page 111) on a regular basis.
- A good way to balance out estrogen and progesterone is to drink two cups of mint tea for fourteen days and then two cups of chamomile for day for fourteen days. The peppermint supports the first half of the menstrual cycle, and the chamomile the latter half.

If you suffer regularly from amenorrhea or late periods, it would be better for you to think in terms of a more holistic treatment instead of simply trying to bring on your period. Consult an herbalist, or try homeopathic remedies or other alternative medicines. Drinking sage and red raspberry leaf teas on a regular basis can help improve this condition, as they help tone the uterus and ovaries. Before trying any of the above methods, we urge women to first make sure they are not with child, as that could result in a miscarriage.

MENORRHAGIA OR EXCESSIVE FLOW

Red raspberry leaves are best as they do not stop you from bleeding, but rather help regulate your flow. Start using them once a week before your period is due and continue throughout menstruation. Repeat if necessary.

The following all help reduce excessive menstrual flow:

- Vitamin C.
- Vitamin T (sesame seeds, sesame butter).

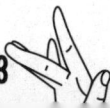

- Bioflavonoids (buckwheat, the skin of citrus fruits, grapes, cherries, blackberries).
- Consider yarrow (page 118) or shepard's purse if flow is excessive and prolonged. Drinking two to three cups per day or two droppersful of tincture four times per day for three days.

DYSMENORRHEA OR PAINFUL PERIODS

Most of us experience sensations ranging from mild discomfort to excruciating pain during menstruation. We get cramps before, during and after our periods. Medical science tells us that to suffer is part of being a woman. But we know this isn't true. Sexually transmitted infections (STIs) are sometimes responsible for pain, but most of the time cramps are caused by inflammation, swelling and tension in the cervix and uterus.

STIs are possible when there is any type of genital contact. This includes gonorrhea, chlamydia, syphillus, genital warts and herpes simplex 1 which is displayed as cold sores on the mouth. The virus HIV is another disease that can be contracted by sexual activity, as can hepatitis.

What To Do:

- Avoid salt, sugar, processed foods (including white sugar, white flour, and white bread) and caffeine (one week prior to your menses).
- Eat foods high in potassium every day- bananas, dry fruits, melons, oranges, carrots, leafy green vegetables and potatoes, as well as foods high in magnesium- nuts, seeds, avocados, leafy green vegetables, fish, and yogurt.

- Eat organic dark green vegetables and oranges for vitamin A (it reduces tension).
- Eat oatmeal, broccoli, parsley (which can be taken as infusion), Brazil nuts, almonds, and seaweed for their high calcium content (which eliminates cramps). Seaweed (kelp in particular) can be taken in tablet form.
- Hot baths, a hot water bottle placed on the lower abdomen, smoking a joint, vigorous or light exercise, and orgasms all help relieve tension, cramping and pain.
- Yarrow (page 118) taken in capsule form, tinctures or infusions provides very good results. Begin one week before your period and continue throughout its duration.
- Ginger (page 105) infusions rapidly relieve cramps. You can also chew the fresh root. Take as needed to relieve pain.
- Red raspberry leaf tea (page 111) works well to alleviate cramps but must be taken regularly (over a period of months). It is mild and can be used for long-term treatment.
- Consider crampbark & valerian (page 116) tea or tincture.
- Magnesium cell salts have worked wonders to alleviate cramps, six pellets under the tongue every twenty minutes until the pain has subsided. These are cell salts—not to be confused with homeopathic pellets.
- Get an Arvigo abdominal massage. This external technique helps to realign a mal-positioned uterus which may be the cause of the discomfort and PMS.

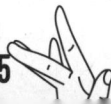

LOVE IN THE AGE OF STIs

There are many simple ways to reduce your risk of contracting a sexually transmitted infection (STI).

What You Need to Know:

- Blood (including menstrual blood), sperm and seminal fluid have the highest concentrations of the virus.
- Vaginal secretions have lower concentrations but can also transmit the disease.
- Vaginal infections such as fungus, yeast, and chlamydia can also increase the risk of transmission.
- Condyloma or herpes are also means of transmission.
- Some cases have been attributed to the ingestion of vaginal secretions, sperm, and breast milk.
- Tears and saliva have little to no traces of the virus, unless they contain blood.
- It is recommended to avoid brushing your teeth before and after a sexual encounter as it can cause bleeding.
- Never share unsterilized needles or syringes (tattoos, piercings). There are needle exchanges at prevention centers and effective ways of cleaning needles or syringes.
- Sex toys (dildos, vibrators...) must be disinfected or covered with a condom before they can be shared.

WHAT YOU NEED TO DO:

- Communicate: Talk with your partner(s) about STIs, sexual health, and prevention prior to sexual activity. Communication encourages trust and respect among partners and helps reduce risks and ensures that you truly like this person.

- Get Tested: When you have had sexual contact with another person who in turn has had sex with anyone else, you begin to run a risk. Testing can help you learn whether you may have contacted an STI, as many STIs are not noticeable until it's too late. Some STD/STIs are not detectable through testing for anywhere from a few weeks to a few months.

- Protect Yourself: Condoms work well in stopping most STIs from being passed from an infected partner to another when they are used immediately, consistently, and correctly every time a person has oral, vaginal, or anal sex.

- Learn about vaccines: Currently, vaccines are available to protect against infection with HPV, hepatitis A, and hepatitis B.

- Decisions made about sex while sober are often more sustainable in the long run.

- Dental dams are squares of plastic used during oral sex to protect the vagina or the anus. They can be replaced by a condom cut length wise or thick saran wrap. Always use water-based lubricants with latex products (no vaseline or other petroleum-based jellies, which disintegrate latex).

- Wear protective gloves for all vaginal or anal penetration with your hands if you have the slightest cut or sore.

- Keep in mind that monogamy is not the same thing as safe sex. If you think you are at risk or if you want to

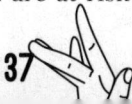

have a child, it's a good idea to get tested. Always request an anonymous test.

If you are sexually active with men who don't want to wear condoms, ask whose interest they have in mind and remind yourself that no fuck is worth risking your life for. Remember that women are 18 percent more likely to be infected with HIV by men than the other way around.

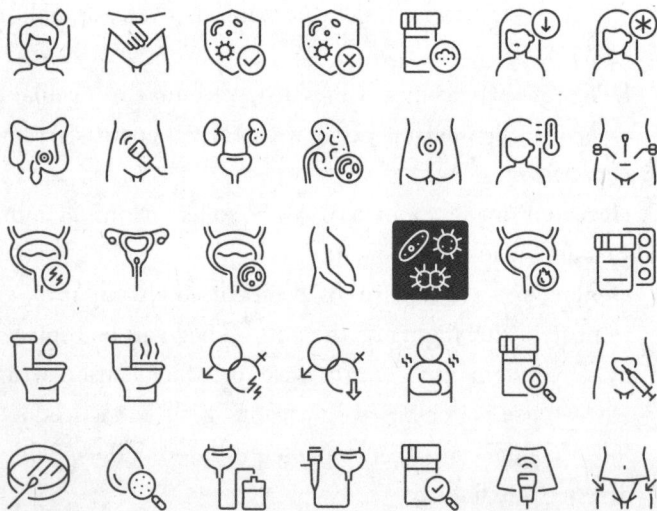

REFERENCES

FOR MORE INFORMATION ABOUT THE DANGERS OF USING BLEACHED TAMPONS AND PADS (AS WELL AS EXCELLENT REFERENCES FOR ALTERNATIVES), CONSULT:

Whitewash by Liz Armstrong and Adrienne Scott. 1992. Harper Collins.

The Doctor's Case Against the Pill. By Barbara Seaman. 1980. Doubleday.

Our Bodies, Ourselves. Boston Women's Health Collective

Take Back Your Life: A Wimmin's Guide to Alternative Healthcare. By Alicia non Grata. Profane Existence Collective.

FOR FURTHER READING:

Susie Sexpert's Lesbian Sex World. By Susie Bright. Cleiss Press. 1990.

The Invisible Epidemic: The Story of Women and Aids. Gena Corea. Harper Perennial.

Making It. By Cindy Patton.

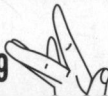

35 YEARS OF FERTILITY

We ovulate every 28 days. That's 15 to 20 times per year and at least 300 menstrual cycles in a lifetime... For those of us who sleep with men, that's thousands of opportunities for getting pregnant. It's normal to change your partners, mind, and methods. It's normal to abort. It's normal to freak out!

These things make it even harder on us:

- Men's indifference, and their ignorance about their own fertility- men are fertile all the time, and we're ultimately the ones who have to deal with it.
- The added responsibility of contraception and protection (against the HIV virus and STIs) which women have to take on themselves.
- The stress which results from having to constantly educate men about taking responsibilities for their bodies... and ours.

It can seem bleak at times, but keep in mind that lovers come and go. Your body is yours for the long haul. Be good to yourself above all. If someone tries to persuade you otherwise, ask yourself whose interests they've got in mind. Our attitudes towards sex have changed. They've had to— it's a matter of survival.

Safe sex is essential and condoms offer the advantage of protecting against both the HIV retro-virus and unwanted pregnancies. Many of us have found

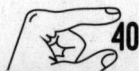

"enforcing" safe sex with our lovers hard. It's a drag listening to guys whine about condoms being uncomfortable or unsexy. It's even more of a drag being in conflict with the person you want to fuck, especially when you'd rather be fucking than arguing.

THE CENTER FOR DISEASE CONTROL'S 2022 REPORT

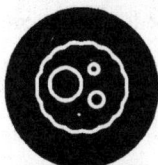

1.6 million
CASES OF CHLAMYDIA
6.2% decrease since 2018

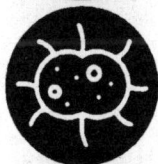

648,056
CASES OF GONORRHEA
11% increase since 2018

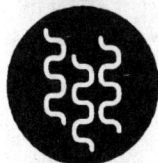

207,255
CASES OF SYPHILIS
80% increase since 2018

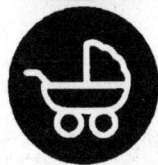

3,755
CASES OF SYPHILIS AMONG NEWBORNS
183% increase since 2018

COMPLETE REPORT AT CDC.GOV/STD

CHECK YOUR MUCUS

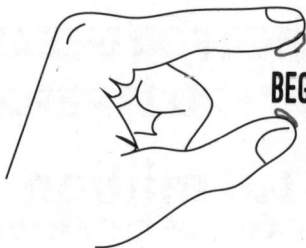

BEGINNING MUCUS:
STICKY, BREAKS
WHEN STRETCHED

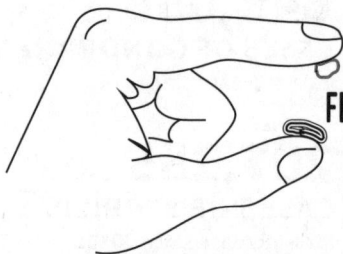

FERTILE MUCUS:
WHITE OR CREAM
COLORED, THICK TO
SLIGHTLY STRETCHY

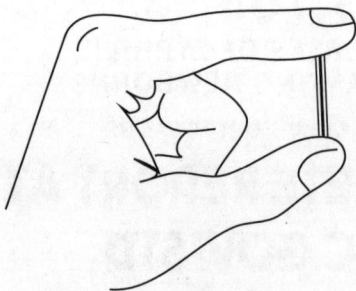

MOST FERTILE MUCUS:
STRETCHY, COLOR IS
SIMILAR TO A RAW EGG
WHITE

TEMPERATURE AND CERVICAL MUCUS CHARTING

Dates covered _____ Cycle number: _____

Cycle day	1	2	3	4	5	6	7	8	9	10	11	12	13	14	15	16	17	18	19	20	21	22	23	24	25	26	27	28	29	30	31	32	33	34	35	36	37	38	39	40
Date																																								
Day of week																																								
Time																																								

BASAL BODY TEMPERATURE (°F)

99.0
98.9
98.8
98.7
98.6
98.5
98.4
98.3
98.2
98.1
98.0
97.9
97.8
97.7
97.6
97.5
97.4
97.3
97.2
97.1
97.0

| CM type | | | | | | | | | | | | | | | | | | | | | | | | | | | | | | | | | | | | | | | | |
| Sex | | | | | | | | | | | | | | | | | | | | | | | | | | | | | | | | | | | | | | | | |

CM types: P=period, D=dry, S=sticky rice, E=egg whites   Notes:

HELPFUL HINTS IN CASE YOU DON'T FOLLOW THIS LINE:

- Never assume you're infertile because you've never gotten pregnant when you have hardly used contraceptives, even if over a long period of time.
- Avoid The Pill; try to opt for alternative methods of contraception: condoms, cervical cap, or diaphragm. While they may seem tedious to use, these methods offer the advantage of not disturbing your body's natural cycle. Take time to get to know your fertile periods by observing your cervical mucus and other signs of ovulation.

It's important to figure out whether your cycle is regular or not, and to understand how it works. Don't worry if it takes you a while to figure it out. Your menstrual cycle is like a good friend—you get to know it better over time. This is a step toward reproductive freedom and the reappropriation of control over our bodies. You may also find it useful to chart your periods on a menstrual calendar. It may be necessary to get your ovaries (et cetera) in better shape: see "Hormonal Imbalance" on page 80 or "Cleansing Your Genitals" on page 82. Red raspberry leaf (page 111) is excellent for toning the uterus and ovaries.

Your vaginal mucus (or discharge) changes during the monthly cycle, and during ovulation it takes on very specific characteristics which allow a woman to know if she is ovulating or not. A sort of "mucus microscope" is available, to check if your cervical mucus is fertile or not. The microscope makes it easier to identify the various properties of your mucus. If you have a microscope, practicing this is easy.

Many health food stores sell them; however they run fairly high in price. It is not uncommon for women living together to all pitch in and share a microscope for the household, but it is also possible to examine without a microscope. Consult the references listed below to find out more about identifying the characteristics of your mucus.

Make sure to read up on this subject and get to know your cycle while using a reliable method of birth control, to make sure if you can tell if your mucus is fertile or not.

Another natural way to predict your fertility is temperature charting, measuring your basal body temperature and cervical mucus to learn your body's patterns and predict ovulation. You can determine when you are fertile or not and can have sex based on whether or not you want to conceive. Because every woman's cycle is different, your chart may differ from a friend's or even from month to month. Start by buying a basal thermometer from most any drugstore.

1. Fill in the dates and days of the week that correspond to the beginning of your period as day one.

2. Each day, take your temperature with the thermometer and check your cervical mucus. Mark your temperature on the chart and record what your cervical mucus looks like. Connect the dots to see how your basal temperature fluctuates from day to day.

4. During your next cycle, complete the chart again and see whether you ovulate with the same frequency. With months

of data, you should see a pattern that will help you predict when you ovulate.

5. If you ovulate on or near the same day in each cycle, you know when to have sex. If your ovulation varies, look for other patterns—for example, when you're about to ovulate, you have two or three days of egg white cervical mucus and then your temperature takes a little dip before rising the next day.

6. Having sex during your most fertile period has the best chance of conceiving. Your most fertile period is about five days long: from three days before ovulation until one day after.

Check out the research and techniques of Aviva Steiner and Reuma Cohen, two women working in Isreal who have developed a method based on using yoga and exercise to inhibit the implantation of the egg in the uterus, and therefore bring on menstrauation.

MORE INFORMATION

Our Bodies, Ourselves by the Boston Women's Health Book Collective: this is a good resource on women's health issues in general; this most recent edition has been expanded to include information on the mucus method and other alternatives to chemical contraceptives and medicines.

Taking Charge of Your Fertility, 10th Anniversary Edition: The Definitive Guide to Natural Birth Control, Pregnancy Achievement, and Reproductive Health. 2006 by Toni Weschler
"Celebrating 10 years of helping hundreds of thousands of women achieve pregnancy, avoid pregnancy naturally, and gain better control of their health and lives...this book provides answers to all these questions, plus amazing insights into a woman's body. Weschler thoroughly explains the empowering Fertility Awareness Method..."

Honoring Our Cycles: A Natural Family Planning Workbook 2006 by Katie Singer

AFTER A RISKY SEXUAL ENCOUNTER

(These are not methods of birth control and should not be used on a regular basis)

If you do have unprotected sex, or if the condom breaks, the following methods can help prevent an unwanted pregnancy. Keep in mind these recipes are not miraculous, and if conception has indeed taken place they often only work 20-30 percent of the time. Again—for success, begin a day or two before your menses is scheduled to begin.

- In the first moments following risky sex (or if a condom breaks), insert one non-chewable Vitamin C tablet (ideally a 500 milligram tablet) into the vagina. The acidity will change the pH-balance in the vagina and prevent sperm from staying alive. Dosage: one to two tablets inserted into the vagina every twelve hours, for three days. This may burn or cause vaginal irritation; in this case, follow the yogurt treatment (see "Yeast Infections" on page 70).
- Take high dosages of Vitamin C orally (see "A Simple Way of Bringing on Your Period" on page 49). This is a good method to use when you're traveling, or as an emergency method.
- Wild carrot seed (page 117) can be used to avoid unwanted pregnancies by preventing the fertilized egg from attaching itself to the uterine wall. Dosage: 1 teaspoon of seeds every day, starting at the time of ovulation or immediately after unsafe sex during the fertile period.Some women take the seeds for one week,

others until the bleeding begins. You can chew on the seeds, take them in a glass of water or juice, or swallow them in gelatin capsules. Make sure that the seeds you buy have not been chemically treated, as this destroys their effectiveness.

A SIMPLE WAY OF BRINGING ON YOUR PERIOD

(If you suspect an unwanted pregnancy)

This recipe should not be used on a regular basis, nor as a method of contraception. It is easy to prepare, costs almost nothing, and it is not known to have side effects. The best time to begin the treatment is on the day that you were supposed to begin menstruating (or the next day).

The treatment lasts three days.

1. Insert a sprig of fresh parsley (page 110) as far as possible into the vagina. Change the parsley every twelve hours. When soft, it may be difficult to remove, but this is not dangerous.

2. At the same time, drink parsley infusions (see page 110 for infusion). Drink 4 oz. every three hours for two to three days.

3. During these three days, take high dosages of Vitamin C orally. The ideal dosage is 500 milligrams every hour (6000 mg per day) for up to six days. Vitamin C can bring on menstruation even three weeks after a "late" period. You can begin taking Vitamin C orally immediately after unsafe sex. If the treatment is successful for you, then you should start to bleed within two or three days. You should know that:

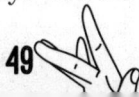

- You may have cramps when you first start to bleed; take ginger infusions (page 105) as needed.
- Chances of this method working are lower for women who regularly take Vitamin C.

This treatment is not advised for women with kidney problems.

HOW TO BRING ON A PERIOD USING EMMENAGOGUES

These methods are not to be used as contraceptives. The recipes here use more concentrated combinations of herbs and are designed to induce a miscarriage. These plants can be used if you wish to abort naturally, but must be used in the manner indicated here. We provide these recipes knowing that only a few women will be able to use them under their optimal conditions.

It's important to know that the earlier you use these herbs, the more effective they'll be, but one condition is absolutely necessary: you have to be at the end of your cycle. This means that they will not work right after ovulation, as it is not possible to eliminate the fertilized egg before it has adhered to the uterine wall. Some herbs such as wild carrot seed can be used to prevent the fertilized egg from attaching itself to the uterine wall (see page 48).

You should begin drinking the teas the night before menstruation is to begin; on that day, or up to six days afterwards—but not later! You may want to have a pregnancy test to verify whether you are really pregnant or not. These plants are not toxic, but keep in mind that if they cause a miscarriage, they are certainly able to damage an embryo. You can use these recipes if you are sure that you can obtain a medical abortion if the herbs do not work. If you are sure you are pregnant, make an appointment for an abortion and then cancel if these recipes succeed.

If you know you are pregnant and are sure that you want to terminate the pregnancy, act as quickly as possible. Women who are aware of their cycles have the greatest chances of success. These recipes are not miraculous, but if you do them early enough, chances of succeeding are fairly good.

Use only one of the following two recipes.

Emmenagogue recipe #1
1. Infuse:
- 1/2 fl. ounce (14 grams) of motherwort (page 109)
- 1/2 (14 gr.) of mugwort (page 109) in 2 or 3 cups of boiling water; steep covered on low heat for twenty minutes and strain.
2. Make a decoction of 1 fl. ounce (28 gr.) of blue cohosh root (page 98) in 2 cups of cold water. Simmer on low heat for twenty minutes (covered) and strain.

INGREDIENTS: MOTHERWORT, MUGWORT, GOLDENSEAL ROOT, BLUE COHOSH ROOT, FRESH GINGER ROOT

3. Mix the infusion (from step one) and the decoction (from step two) together.

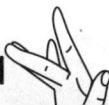

Dosage:

Drink hot, one-fourth of a cup, four to five times per day, or drink a total of one and one-half cups per day, taking a small amount every hour.

In addition:

Take two goldenseal root capsules (page 106) three times a day; chew on fresh ginger and/or drink as many ginger infusions (page 105) as possible.

Keep in mind:

- The infusion tastes rather awful; add honey.
- Stop taking the mixture as soon as you start bleeding, or after taking it for four days with no results.
- Most women should begin menstruating within 48 hours or so after beginning treatment.
- You should know that these herbs can cause contractions and/or dizziness; lots of rest is advised. They may also induce nausea and/or vomiting; eat lightly.
- Do these treatments with a friend. They can check your progress, give support, massage, keep you sane, etc.
- Practice has shown that the more advanced the pregnancy, the more severe the side effects, and therefore not recommended. Schedule for an abortion consult.
- This treatment should not be done more than six days after a missed period. See "Side Effects" below.

Emmenagogue Recipe #2

INGREDIENTS:

2 tablespoons dried blue cohosh root
3 tablespoons dried pennyroyal leaves

2 tablespoons dried tansy leaves and flowers (or leaves from the plant in flower)

1. Put the blue cohosh root (page 98) in 6 cups of water and bring it to a boil. Add the remaining herbs as soon as it boils, cover, and remove from heat.

2. Let it steep for at least 30 minutes.

3. Strain out the herbs and reheat (do not boil) before using.

Dosage:
One cup, as hot as possible, every three to four hours for no more than five days. Drinking this recipe while sitting in a hot bath increases its effectiveness.

Side Effects For Emmenagogues
Contractions, dizziness, nausea, vomiting

Important: Even though complications are very, very rare, if you experience any of the following symptoms after using one of these recipes, go to a hospital immediately: extremely severe nausea, very high fever (103-104 degrees F.), hemorrhaging (soaking through more than two pads an hour for over four hours). In the case of an incomplete miscarriage, a dilation and curettage (D&C—or scraping of the uterine wall) may be necessary. Emmenagogue recipes numbers one and two should **not** be used together.

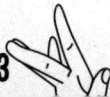

You can take ginger infusions (page 105) or eat fresh ginger root while using emmenagogue recipe found on the previous page.

OTHER EMMENAGOGUES

Tansy leaves and flowers (page 114) can be taken in infusion, or tincture (page 89) to bring on a miscarriage. This plant helps stimulate menstrual flow.

Dosage: One cup of infusion every two hours or 10-15 drops of tincture in warm water every two hours.

THINGS YOU SHOULD KNOW

*   Make sure you choose good-quality dried herbs from a reliable source.
*   Visualization and meditation help when using emmenagogues: imagine the egg being dislodged from the uterus and then expelled. Having someone massage or press down on your lower abdomen can help stimulate uterine contractions and induce menstruation.
*   Alcohol, sugar, nicotine and caffeine all interfere with the body's ability to absorb herbs. Try to minimize your intake of these substances while taking these treatments.
*   Drink lots and lots of water when using any of the recipes and herbs listed above. Herbs can be hard on the liver and kidneys and one must be well hydrated in order to flush them out.

Do not, under any circumstances, exceed the recommended dosages. Once again, even though complications are very, very rare, if you do experience any of the following symptoms after using these recipes, go to a hospital immediately: extremely severe nausea, very high fever (103-104 F.), or hemorrhaging (soaking through more than two pads an hour for over four hours).

In the case of an incomplete miscarriage, a dilation and curettage (D&C—or scraping of the uterine wall) may be necessary.

REFERENCES

The Wise Woman Herbal for the Childbearing Year. By Susun S. Weed (Ash Tree Publishing, Woodstock, New York) : while designed for women who want to have a baby, the first section deals with herbal methods for avoiding and terminating an unwanted pregnancy. And should you ever change your mind and decide you would like to conceive, this book is a very helpful guide to a healthy pregnancy and childbirth.

Herbal Healing for Women 1993 by Rosemary Gladstar "For centuries women have turned to herbs to cope with a wide variety of health problems and conditions. Comprehensive and easy-to-use, Herbal Healing for Women explains how to create remedies—including teas, tinctures, salves, and ointments—for the common disorders that arise in the different cycles of a woman's life. Covering adolescence, childbearing years, pregnancy and childbirth, and menopause, Rosemary Gladstar teaches how herbs can be used to treat the symptoms of conditions such as acne, PMS, morning sickness, and hot flashes."

Botanical Medicine for Women's Health 2009 by Aviva Romm
"A comprehensive resource of medical and herbal interventions related to women's health issues, Botanical Medicine for Women's Health provides a unique combination of traditional and modern scientific data on herbal medicine. Written by Aviva Romm, MD, an experienced herbalist, physician, and midwife, this guide blends a clinician-sensitive and patient-centered approach to women's health issues. Coverage of menstrual health, fertility, breast conditions, and more makes this an essential resource for everyday practice."

Take Back Your Life. A Wimmin's Guide to Alternative Heath Care. By Alicia non Grata.

FIBROID OF LABIUM MAJUS

(ONE OF THE LABIUM MAGORA)

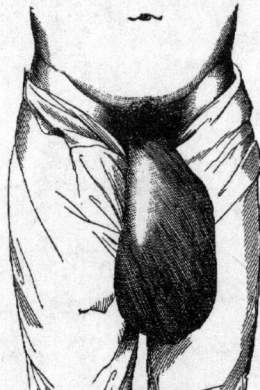

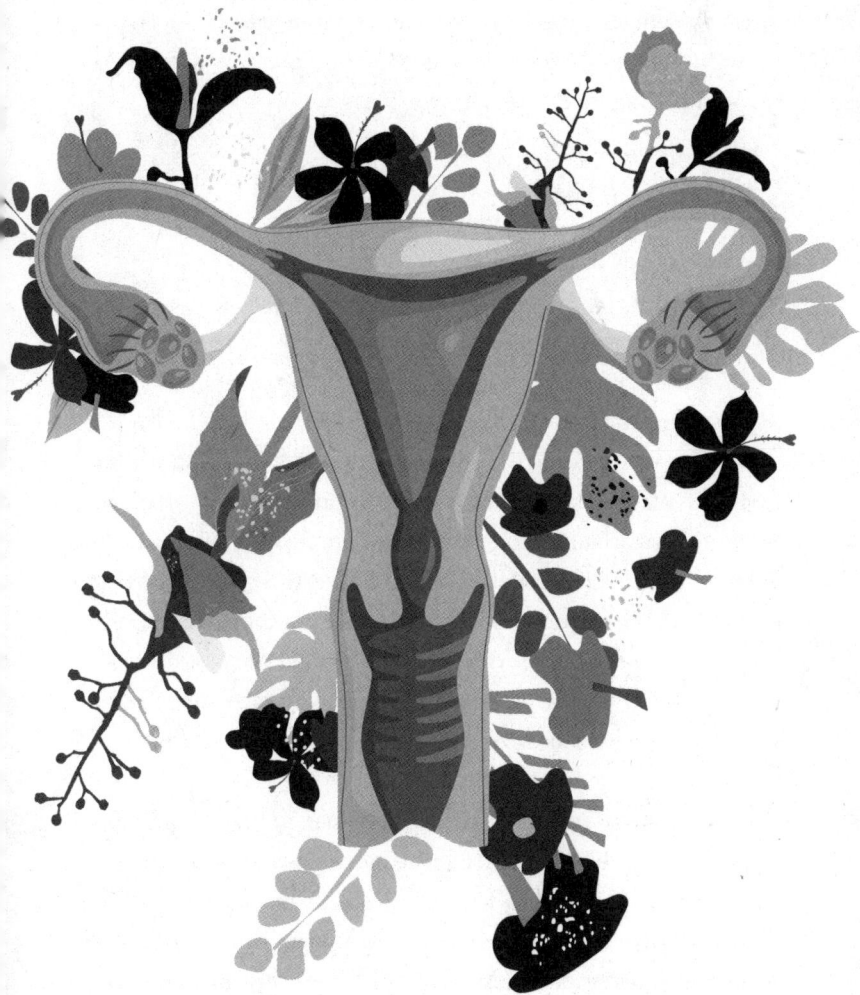

STIs & OTHER ALIENS

It's a good idea to go for regular gynecological check-ups; if a problem is diagnosed, you can then decide not to treat it with chemical pills or creams. While current standards recommend at PAP every three years for women aged 21–45, if you experience any new symptoms that are not your normal, an exam should be considered. Pap tests ensure that all is well with a woman's cervix, in an effort to prevent cervical cancer or other complications.

Chemical antibiotics are not advised (especially if you've already taken them a number of times) because they tend to weaken the immune system (and your defenses against other illnesses in addition to the one you are treating). Though you may want to avoid medical treatment, clinics offer tests for the problems and STIs mentioned in this section. Some of their symptoms are very similar, and it's best to determine which STI you have before treating yourself with herbal remedies. Certain STIs such as gonorrhea can result in pelvic inflammatory disease (PID), infertility and other complications if left untreated. If these treatments do not work for you, be sure to see a good gynecologist for medical treatment.

Human Papilloma Virus (HPV) is another infection that is frequently transmitted through skin-to-skin or sexual contact. It is believed to lead to cervical cancers and should be dealt with. People with HPV do not exhibit symptoms so get tested regularly. A vaccine is available that protects against 70 percent of the types of HPV that cause cancer, but long term studies on its effectiveness or possible side effects are yet to be determined.

The treatments suggested here are plant-based: some of them are natural antibiotics that strengthen the immune system to combat disease or infection. Their effectiveness is high as these plants cleanse the body while diminishing the chances of reinfection. Even if you're pretty sure you've gotten rid of the infection, get a test after completing an herbal treatment just in case you still have undetected symptoms.

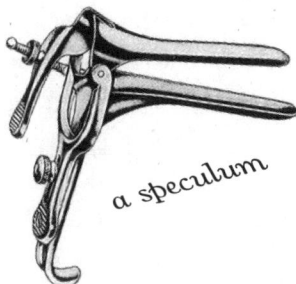

a speculum

Get a hold of a speculum. Ask your gynecologist; if they use disposable ones, they may be able to give you one. Examine yourself with a mirror and a flashlight. It's always worth it to visit a new part of your body! Smell, taste, touch. You'll quickly be able to tell what's not quite right. Most infections can be detected before symptoms such as vaginal discharge and itching appear. Once you become familiar with the normal, healthy state of your vagina, a vaginal exam using a speculum allows you to detect the first signs of an infection. You'll be able to spot parts of the vagina or cervix that are redder than usual, or notice small red marks on the cervix. You can also get together with friends and check each

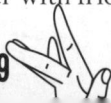

other out. This is a good way to compare and exchange experience. The references provided at the end of this chapter provide sources of information on self-examinations.

Most people prefer to treat STDs with antibiotics; it is generally the easiest way to dispel the infection. However, keep in mind that if you decide to take chemical antibiotics, you may be put at risk for a yeast infection. If this happens to be the case, eat lots of plain natural yogurt (the kind with active bacteria) to restore the vagina's natural pH balance. Avoid acidic fruits and sugar. Vaginal yogurt tablets or acidophilus tablets can also prevent yeast infections. Or, with the help of a speculum, you can insert yogurt into the vagina using a small spoon or a large "baby syringe" (one that doesn't have a needle—page 92). Red raspberry leaf tea (page 111) or yarrow (page 118) can be used to restore equilibrium to the genitals after taking antibiotics. Take these for a month or more.

When consulting a physician or gynecologist, it's not a bad idea to get a second opinion and find out if it's absolutely necessary to treat your condition with chemical medicine (unfortunately, sometimes it is). Ask about alternatives— sympathetic doctors will understand your concerns. Most doctors push antibiotics on us for even the most minor problems and pharmaceutical companies make a huge profit from this. We don't have to support them. Herbal medicine has proved itself for centuries... And the choice is yours.

If you have an infection or STI, it's important that both you and your sexual partner(s) follow these treatments as STIs are easily passed back and forth—this will help you avoid reinfection after completing a treatment. Men can heal themselves with these treatments by taking the herbs in infusion or tincture form (refer to specific notes in text). Keep in mind that practicing safe sex can prevent the transmission of most STIs, and reduces the risk of reinfection after a treatment.

CRABS

Everyone, even small children, can get crabs. They are tiny insect-like creatures that lay their eggs in clothes, sofas, bedding, and carpets. Crabs cannot survive for more than 24 to 48 hours without a host to feed off of. It's very important to destroy their eggs as well.

SYMPTOMS

They itch! The itchiness is concentrated to the genital region and other hairy areas of the body (even eyebrows). They are small, and their eggs look like tiny brown dots at the base of the hair.

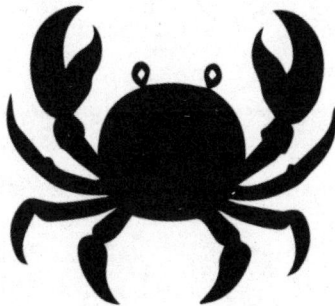

WHAT TO DO

Clothes, towels, and bed linen should be washed in hot water and machine dried on a high setting. Rugs and carpets should be "quarantined" (kept out of contact) for ten to fifteen days, depending on the severity of the invasion. Thyme (page 115), red thyme (more potent), or lavender essential oil (page 107) diluted in olive oil (2 to 3 teaspoons of essential oil for every 5 fl. ounces or 142 ml. of olive oil) can be rubbed onto the infected areas (skin and hair) and left on all night. Wash off with soap. Repeat as needed. If it's especially bad, apply three times a day or more. Drink thyme infusions (infusion recipe on page 115).

SCABIES

Scabies are tiny parasites that live and feed under the outermost layer of our skin, digging long furrows where the female lays her eggs.

SYMPTOMS

After an incubation period of several weeks, acute itchy spots will appear during the night. Scratching accentuates and spreads the red lines.

Hands, between the fingers, wrists, elbows, armpits, the genital area and ankles are where scabies tend to hang out.

WHAT TO DO

Same treatment as for crabs, rub affected areas.

GENITAL WARTS

While they are often called venereal warts, you don't necessarily get them through sexual contact. Whether it's on your cervix or on your finger, a wart is a wart. Warts can disappear without treatment but it's best to take action early. Their presence is said to reflect some sort of deficiency (vitamin, nutritional, etc.). Warts will often appear during pregnancy or with vaginal infections and tend to disappear afterwards. Genital warts often resemble ordinary warts and sometimes appear to be shaped like a rooster's crown with white tips. They can grow internally and externally, in the anal and genital areas.

WHAT TO DO

Doctors treat warts with a toxic cream, Podophyllin, or by harsher methods: electrolysis, liquid nitrogen, laser therapy, or surgery. Ask for documentation.

A home remedy you can use before seeking medical intervention:

Treat your immune system: three weeks of echinacea root (page 103) followed by one week of goldenseal root (page 106).Do the treatment for four weeks; repeat if necessary after a three week break. You can take tinctures instead of infusions, as they are much more convenient for long-term treatments.

You can also rub a clove of garlic (page 104), cut in half, directly onto the warts (if they are accessible). Beware- this may burn! Try to do this two or three times a day for several months, and you should have positive results.

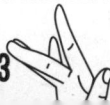

Fresh chickweed (page 101) is very effective in dissolving warts over an extended period of several months. Eat the fresh plant or make an infusion (page 86). The only way to get fresh chickweed is to pick it yourself—it grows all over the city and countryside—see page 77 for things you should know about picking your own herbs.

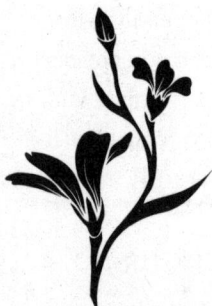

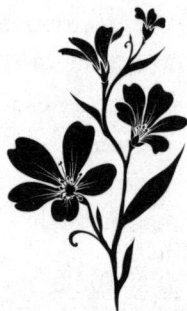

TAKE NOTE:

Warts can be easily spread through hand-to-genital and genital-to-genital contact. Some people are more resistant to warts than others— you should take precautions: use a condom or dental dam if you or your partner is infected; try to wash your hands before sexual contact, or (this is a tough one) reduce hand-to-genital contact.

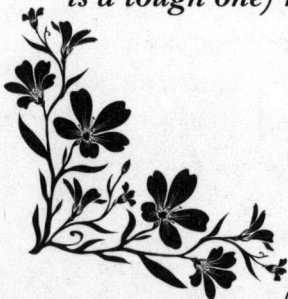

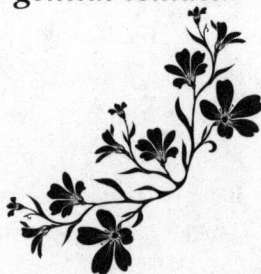

HERPES

Herpes simplex-II is very similar to simplex-I (cold sores on the mouth and lips). It is said to affect only the genital region, but it can develop on any part of the body. The most common means of transmission is genital-to-genital contact, though herpes can also be passed from one person to another during mouth-to-genital or hand-to-genital contact. Lesions will appear between two to ten days after exposure, or more, accompanied by a fever and flu-like symptoms. Some women will experience an outbreak instead of the flu, before or after menstruating, and when under stress. Herpes is a virus, which means that it lives in your system and can reappear. Women who have herpes may want to avoid chocolate, nuts, caffeine, sugar, and alcohol in order to prevent outbreaks.

WHAT TO DO

If breakouts are an infrequent recurrence (once or twice a year), take goldenseal root capsules (page 106) at the onset of the outbreak and for two weeks afterwards. Repeat if the outbreak reoccurs.

VERY FREQUENT RECURRENCE:

The immune system must be treated for a long time (up to one year). Take echinacea root (page 103) until the problem is gone. Use a tincture (page 89) to facilitate absorption. Another good remedy for herpes is garlic, taken in capsules or tablets. Take a high dose (twelve capsules) at the onset of an outbreak (characterized as a tingling sensation), and then three capsules every four hours for three days. It is recommended that you take a dosage of four to six capsules a day for up to one year after the initial treatment. Kyolic garlic tablets are suggested as they are easily digested and have no odor.

DURING THE OUTBREAK:

Take baths, walk around naked (fresh air dries out sores). Apply white clay and let it dry several times a day; clay heals and helps relieve pain. Rest. Relax.

Diet:

- Grapes are advised for their antiviral properties, concentrated in their skins.

- Brewer's yeast (in tablets). Reminder: this is not advised for people who are prone to yeast infections.

- Vitamin C, Vitamin A, Vitamin E.

- Take 1000mg of lysine at first tingling sensation of outbreak. Take every hour for 24–48 hours which often cuts it off at the pass. Do not exceed two weeks with treatment.

- Try to understand what triggers an attack: stress, depression, which foods, which clothes, menstruation, etc... And try to avoid what you can.

- Avoid coffee, chocolate, nuts, sugar, and alcohol.

- Take lots of garlic (page 86) fresh and in tablets or capsules.

For more information about herpes, consult: *Our Bodies, Ourselves* by the Boston Women's Collective.

BLADDER & URINARY INFECTIONS

SYMPTOMS

Having to pee all the time, pressure in the bladder, feeling the urge to pee but nothing comes out (or maybe just two or three drops), blood in the urine, dark urine with a strong odor. Be careful, these signs may be indicative of a more serious infection such as Pelvic Inflammatory Disease (PID). If fever starts or pain in the kidneys that is similar to menstrual cramps is felt, pyelonephritis is likely. Check with a doctor if you're not sure.

CAUSES

Imbalances in the intestinal bacteria, wiping from back to front, nylon underwear, chemical foams, food allergies or irritant, sexual positions, stress, cold, any type of vaginal penetration or contact—including anal penetration followed by vaginal penetration—done without cleaning the fingers, penis, or sex toys in between.

WHAT TO DO

For those consistently suffering from this type of infection, drinking cranberry juice daily is a must. Drink a 16 fl. ounce glass hourly at the first signs of an infection. This will usually stop it in a couple of hours. Continue drinking 16 fl. ounces of cranberry juice at least twice daily for prevention. If nothing but water is available, drink a 16 fl. ounce glass hourly and make sure you are drinking at least eight glasses a day after that. It also helps to reduce sexual positions that cause rubbing on the urethra.

- Bearberry (page 98) in infusion or tincture is very good. You'll probably feel like your bladder is going to burst, but it's sure to get rid of the infection.
- Take yarrow (page 118) in infusion or tincture (page 89).
- Try a more alkaline diet comprised of fruits, almonds, leeks, turnips and barley.
- Avoid coffee, tea, meat, white flower, sugar, and acid generating foods.
- In addition, take goldenseal capsules (page 106) for two weeks.
- In case of pain, take valerian (page 116) capsules or tincture as needed.

CHLAMYDIA

Chlamydia often occurs without symptoms in many women. Its presence is indicated by an infected cervix with a yellowish color (check with a speculum), a burning sensation when urinating and heavy vaginal discharge. You can also contract chlamydia in your throat during oral sex. If you suspect that you may have contracted chlamydia, or if you're not sure of your symptoms, have a test done. It is an STD that can be treated with one pill if one chooses to use antibiotics, but we like to always include the herbal alternative.

If gone untreated over a long period of time, chlamydia can lead to long-term complications like Pelvic Inflammatory Disease.

WHAT TO DO

Take echinacea (page 103) twice a week for three weeks; taking it as a tincture (page 89) will help facilitate absorption. Eat raw garlic or take garlic capsules (page 104) every day. Do this for one to two months, depending on the severity of the infection. After the treatment has ended have another test done to make sure the infection is really gone.

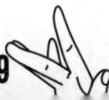

VAGINITIS & VULVITIS

This is a catch-all term for several disorders: yeast infections (candida), trichomonas and gardnarella. These conditions are inflammation of the vagina and vulva; they depend on many factors and are not caused exclusively by sexual intercourse. Spermicide, antibiotics, latex and perfumed soaps can induce vaginitis or vulvitis in certain women. Sensitivity to these and other irritants vary with each and every woman. Specific causes and their treatments follow.

YEAST INFECTIONS AND CANDIDA

This infection is caused by a yeast-like fungus called candida, normally found in the vagina. The vagina usually protects against infection through the production of bacteria which maintain its natural acidity. When the acidity is altered, it allows bacteria such as candida to multiply in large numbers, causing the infection.

Yeast infections are not considered a sexually transmitted disease but they can be transmitted through sexual intercourse. If you have a yeast infection, penetration of any sort (penis, sex toys, fingers) is not recommended (even with a condom) since it can aggravate the irritation. Wash your hands and genitals after any sexual contact with an infected partner as it is very easy to become reinfected through intercourse or hand-to-genital contact.

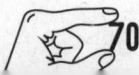

CAUSES

Nervousness, fatigue, pregnancy, heat, a sudden change in your life, a new sexual partner, stress, vitamin B deficiency, eating too much sugar, wearing tight-fitting or synthetic underwear... Antibiotics will often bring on a yeast infection as they wipe out many of the vagina's natural bacteria, allowing candida to reproduce in high numbers.

SYMPTOMS

Thick, cottage-cheesy white discharge with a sweetish odor. Itchiness of the vulva or vagina followed by irritation and swelling of the labia. It gets worse if you scratch.

TREATMENT

Plain natural yogurt is very effective. Insert it with a teaspoon (or a speculum if necessary). Wear a pad as the yogurt will flow out. Make sure to use unpasteurized yogurt containing live lactobacilli. You can also use vaginal yogurt capsules. Acidophillus capsules work even better; but as they are small, you should insert several capsules (two or three) into the vagina. They can be taken orally at the same time. Do this for five to ten days, preferably at night. In a crisis situation use yogurt three to four times a day. "Baby syringes" will work well to insert yogurt and are available in drugstores. Yogurt can also be applied using those gadgets used for inserting spermicide with a diaphragm—they can sometimes be bought separately. Coconut oil has also been found to help with the treatment of yeast infections, as it can explode the centers of candida.

Boric acid capsules work well too. Insert one vaginally each night for seven days.

Or follow the garlic treatments indicated for trichomonas below.

Yeast infections are often asymptomatic in men. Men can get rid of yeast infection by rubbing yogurt and/or garlic on the penis every night for seven to ten days.

FOR TREATING ITCHING

Use 1 teaspoon of baking soda in one cup of water. Apply to the vulva as needed.

DIET

Avoid eating acid-generating foods (citrus fruit, tomatoes, etc.), sugar, and white flour. Eat foods rich in vitamin B (dark leafy vegetables). Eat large quantities of yogurt and raw garlic daily.

TRICHOMONAS

This is a one-cell parasite organism, often transmitted during sexual contact or by humid conditions.
Frequent recurrence after menstruation.

SYMPTOMS

Abundant yellowish discharge, unpleasant "fishy" smell, itching; small red dots on the vaginal walls and on the cervix (visible with a speculum); thread-like secretions, sometimes foamy; irritation around the vulva and opening of the vagina.

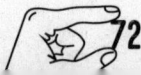

WHAT TO DO

Garlic cloves (page 104) can be inserted into the vagina: try not to nick the clove while peeling it. Wrap it up in a cheesecloth or gauze (you can leave a "tail" which can then be used for easy removal like a tampon), and dip into olive oil or almond oil to avoid irritating the mucous membrane. Change the clove two to three times a day for the first two days and then once in the morning and once at night for five to six days. Men can drink garlic infusions or take garlic tablets.

Or take goldenseal capsules (page 106) orally.
Continue this treatment for two weeks.

Or insert goldenseal capsules into vagina nightly for seven days.

GARDNARELLA

SYMPTOMS

Greyish vaginal discharge with a strong smell.

WHAT TO DO

Same treatment as for Trichomonas.

BACTERIAL INFECTIONS & GONORRHEA

These problems indicate that the immune system has to be seriously treated and built up. Be patient; the treatments can be long. These problems can recur frequently after the first attack; it's better to get rid of them for good.

SYMPTOMS

Light greyish secretions, terrible smell, irritation or itchiness of the vulva. Often occurs without symptoms.

WHAT TO DO

Gonorrhea is another infection that is easily treated by one pill, but an alternative option exists for those who do not feel comfortable with antibiotics.

Echinacea decoction or tincture (page 89 for tincture; page 103 for echinacea) for two to three months, Take valerian (page 96) to relieve discomfort if need be OR echinacea for three weeks followed by goldenseal (page 106) for one week. It is recommended that you take these herbs in tincture form to facilitate their absorption. Take a one week break and repeat the same pattern two more times. Do this with your partner. Valerian (page 116) relieves discomfort if needed.

In case of gonorrhea or syphilis you'd be well advised to consult a naturopath, herbalist or homeopath, and, if necessary, a gynecologist.

Herbs are awesome, but this might be a case for simple antibiotics.

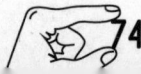

Remember, though you may want to avoid medical treatment, many clinics offer tests for the problems and STIs mentioned in this section. Some of their symptoms are very similar, and it's best to determine which STI you have before treating yourself with herbal remedies. Certain STIs such as gonorrhea can result in Pelvic Inflammatory Disease (PID), infertility, and other complications if left untreated. If these treatments do not work for you, be sure to see a good gynecologist for medical treatment.

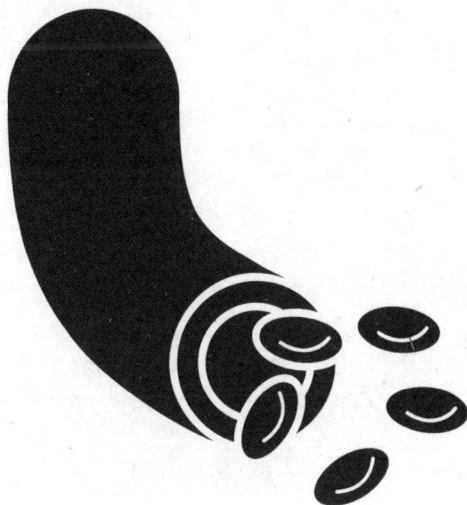

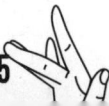

REFERENCES

FOR MORE INFO ON CANDIDA (ESPECIALLY FOR WOMEN WHO ARE PRONE TO YEAST INFECTIONS), CONTACT THE CANDIDA RESEARCH INFORMATION SERVICE AT (416) 832-0789.

For specific symptoms, diagnoses, and information of using a speculum, consult *Our Bodies, Ourselves* by the Boston Women's Health Book Collective.

Herbal Healing for Women 1993 by Rosemary Gladstar

Botanical Medicine for Women's Health 2009 by Aviva Romm

Take Back Your Life: A Wimmen's Guide to Alternative Health Care by Alicia non Grata, published by Profane Existence (available at MicrocosmPublishing.com).

Natural Healing in Gynaecology by Rina Nissim

THE OVARIES & THE UTERUS

OVARIAN PAIN

This usually comes between the tenth and fifteenth day of the cycle (counting from the onset of menstruation). A sharp pain on either or both sides of the lower abdomen means that the egg is being released with difficulty. This can also cause spotting. While there may be internal inflammation, it is usually tension that causes pain.

WHAT TO DO

- Keep a hot water bottle on the lower abdomen.
- Take an infusion of ginger (page 105), red raspberry leaves (page 111), celery seed (page 100), or valerian (page 116) for pain if need be.
- Exercise.
- Improve or modify your diet (see suggestions in the sections "Premenstrual Syndrome" (page 28), and "Dysmennorhea or Painful Periods" (page 34).

OVARIAN CYSTS

Medical science tends to dramatize and often treats them with surgery. Cysts are quite common; for some women they appear regularly throughout the course of their menstrual cycles. Tiny at first, they grow throughout the cycle until eventually decreasing in size. The most common signs are severe pain, urine retention, constipation and discomfort around the anus when shitting.

Cysts that do not go away may require long-term treatment, and even medical attention, as they can become malignant; this is especially true of cervical cysts.

WHAT TO DO

- A diet based on raw vegetables combined with daily exercise encourages cysts to dissolve.

- Red raspberry leaf tea (page 111) taken for three to six months improves the overall state of the ovaries and reduces inflammation of the cysts (because they taste good, raspberry leaves are easily taken over long periods of time).

- If the cysts are really bothering you, take three capsules of cayenne pepper (page 99) every day, as well as infusions of yarrow (page 118) for six weeks, accompanied by infusions or tinctures of red raspberry leaves (page 111). Do this treatment as needed.

- Chickweed (page 101) in tincture form is very effective for dissolving cysts, especially ovarian cysts, when taken over long periods of time.

- Check the quality of your digestion: intestinal problems (such as gas and constipation) are often confused with pain from cysts.

- Apply castor oil packs daily.

- Try an Arvigo uterine massage.

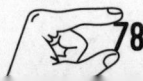

For pain: valerian (page 116) in tincture as needed. If pain persists, see a homeopath, naturopath, or seek medical attention.

FIBROIDS IN THE UTERUS

Most of the time, these are benign, but they do have a tendency to grow larger during the cycle. After menopause the tumors usually diminish or disappear. 20 to 30 percent of women over the age of 30 have fibroid tumors. Sometimes a vigorous exercise program will get rid of them. If the fibroids grow fast, are large, painful, or press on the bladder or colon, they must be surgically removed. Aside from exceptional cases, this does not mean that a hysterectomy is needed, but rather a myectomy: removal of the fibrous tumor itself. Fibroids can also be treated, but it is a rigorous road of herbal teas, tinctures and capsule combining. Consult your local herbalist, naturopath, acupuncturist, or traditional healer.

WHAT TO DO

- Try cleansing your genital organs; refer to page 68.
- Stimulate blood circulations by taking cayenne pepper capsules (page 99) or try this drastic method: sit in a tub of cold water every morning for two to five minutes, or even longer if possible.
- A diet incorporating lots of raw vegetables is recommended. Valerian (page 116) as needed for pain.
- Castor oil packs daily

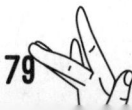

- Arvigo uterine massage
- Moxa on abdomen
- Acupuncture
- Be patient!

VARICOSE VEINS ON THE CERVIX

Visible with a speculum, they are thin, purple, spindly veins which resemble varicose veins on the legs. They tend to be painful before menstruation.

WHAT TO DO

- Cayenne pepper (page 99) for the whole month or the few days before menstruation.
- Vitamin E (nuts, bran, wheat germ) and vitamin C.

HORMONAL IMBALANCE

You may experience a hormonal imbalance due to menopause, taking or getting off of the pill, losing large amounts of weight, serious stress or large intakes of hop products or non-fermented soy in your diet.

Some of these symptoms may be present in women who go off the pill— sometimes for up to 6 months.

HORMONAL IMBALANCES CAN RESULT IN:

- Missed periods
- Unusually long or short periods; unusually light or heavy flow
- An extremely long or short menstrual cycle
- Severe PMS or heavy cramping before or at the onset of menstruation

WHAT TO DO

- Use a combination of licorice root (page 108), red raspberry leaves (page 111) and rosehips (page 112). Make a regular decoction (page 87) using 1/2 ounce licorice (14 gr.) and 1/2 ounce of rose hips in 4 cups of cold water. Make a regular infusion (page 86) using 1 ounce (28 gr.) of red raspberry leaves in 2 or 3 cups of boiling water. Strain and mix the two preparations.
- Use combination of vitex, motherwort, red raspberry and rosehips. Put 4 tablespoons in 1 quart of boiling water and let it steep overnight. Strain in the morning and drink this amount each day for twelve weeks- sip on it all day long, divided up into three cups, drink it hot or cold.
- An herbal tincture of these herbs listed above formulated for you would also prove beneficial. Dosage: one dropperful three times per day.

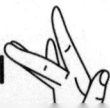

DOSAGE:

1/4 cup, three times a day. Do this treatment for six weeks. Stop for three weeks and start again as needed. An easier way is to use all these plants in tinctures, available in health food stores. Take five to ten drops of each herb tincture two to three times a day. Other, more elaborate treatments are available but are too long to list here.

DIET

Eat seaweed regularly or take in kelp capsules every day.

CLEANSING YOUR GENITALS

The following herbs cleanse our genitals where cysts, adhesions, fibroids, etc. take refuge. This combination of herbs will help in cases of painful, irregular, overly heavy or absent periods and, sometimes, infertility.

WHAT TO DO

- Prepare an infusion (page 86) with yarrow (page 118), red raspberry leaves (page 111), and fresh ginger root (page 105)—grate an inch or two. Use 1 ounce (28 gr.) of red raspberry leaves, 1 ounce of yarrow, and 1 ounce of ginger in 6 to 8 cups of water.
- Dosage: 1/2 cup three times a day. Also take one capsule of cayenne pepper (page 99) three times a day.
- Follow this treatment for six weeks. Considering the fact that cleansing is a slow process (it takes at least as much time to cleanse ourselves as it takes for the system to clog up), stop the treatment for three weeks and start again for six weeks as needed.

- Here again we can make it easier for ourselves by taking the herbs in tincture form (five to ten drops of each plant, two to three times a day); combine this with infusions of ginger or eat the fresh grated root

- For a vaginal steam, mix 3 tablespoons each of lavender (page 107), calendula, basil, and rosemary (page 112). Add to large stock pot filled with boiling water. Set pot under a slatted chair and sit down, having removed all of your clothes from the waist down. Cover lower half of the body and chair with a blanket, trapping heat from the pot inside and funneling the steam up through the slats to the vaginal area. Sit and relax for 30 minutes.

- Drink lots of water with all of these treatments.

Again, other, more elaborate treatments are available but are too long to list here.

FOR FURTHER READING

Des plantes qui querisset by Marie Provost

Wise Woman Herbal for the Childbearing Year by Susun S. Weed

Healing Wise (Wise Woman Herbal Series) 2003 by Susun S. Weed

childbearing-year.com

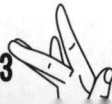

APHRODISIACS

Most of the plants mentioned in this section are spices. They work on the erogenous centers by carrying an intense blood flow to the peripheral organs, which in turn leads to sexual arousal. Because of their strong aroma and the increase in energy provided, spices excite sensoral perceptions.

CINNAMON (STICK OR POWDER FORM)

- Soak 20 grams of cinnamon in 1 liter of sweet wine for ten days and drink two small glasses a day.
- Or simmer 20 grams of cinnamon with a few cloves for fifteen to twenty minutes in 1 liter of good red wine. Sweeten with honey and drink one cup as desired.

GINGER

- Grate a good quantity of the fresh root, add to water and simmer covered for twenty minutes. Drink a small cup after meals. This also improves digestion and helps with nausea or upset stomach.

CLOVES

- Mix half a teaspoon of powdered cloves with honey. (Use it like jam.)
- Or infuse two or three cloves in 1 cup of boiling water. Steep twenty minutes. Drink one to two cups a day.
- Or steep two to three cloves in 1 cup of good hot red wine for a few minutes. Add some lemon rind.cinnamon, and a pinch of nutmeg.

ROSEMARY

- Steep one handful in boiling water. Drink two to three cups everyday.
- Or infuse 50 grams of leaves and branches in 1 liter of dry white wine for ten days. Drink two to three small glasses every day.

SAVORY

- Infuse one handful in boiling water. Drink three cups per day.
- Or for very efficient results, pour four to five drops of savory essential oil on a sugar cube. Take every day or as needed.

CHINESE HERBS

Ginger and royal jelly are also aphrodisiacs and tonics. Available (and less expensive) in Chinese herbal stores, ginseng is used in Chinese medicine to strengthen the elderly and is always used carefully. Seek advice from the salesperson.

Ginseng is commonly used for men; royal jelly for women.

HOW TO PREPARE AND USE HERBS

Preparing herbal tea for taste and pleasure is not the same as preparing herbal infusions and decoctions for medicinal purposes. Avoid using pots, pans and utensils made of aluminum. Go for enameled, stainless steel or glass pots with wooden utensils. Use filtered or spring water for more potent potions.

Note that there are several different ways to prepare infusions, decoctions, tinctures, etc. Opinions on what constitutes an infusion or decoction can vary from one herbal therapist or practitioner to another. What we have chosen to do is to provide the easiest methods of preparation, while ensuring potent and effective treatments. This is good for dried herbs. Use slightly more when they are fresh.

If you want to further explore the subject of plant preparation, consult the Herbal Pharmacy section of either Susun S. Weed's two books, *The Wise Women Herbal: Healing Wise* and *Wise Woman Herbal for the Childbearing Year.* They are excellent.

REGULAR INFUSION FOR MOST FLOWERS, LEAVES, AND STEMS:

A VERY BASIC METHOD

Put 4 tablespoons of herbs, leaves or flowers in 1 quart of boiling water and let it steep overnight. Strain in the morning and drink this amount each day for twelve weeks. You can sip on it all day long, divided up into three cups; drink it hot or cold.

This is good for all herbal parts; roots, bark, flower, seed, and leaves. It can be steeped all together rather than needing to boil some part plants and then add it to an infusion of other plant parts.

ANOTHER METHOD

(This method is more effective as it extracts more of the plant's medicinal properties.)

- Use 2 ounces (two large handfuls) of the plant parts you need per every 4–5 cups of water used (or 1 ounce of plant per 2–3 cups of water).
- Bring the water to a boil. Put the plant material in a mason jar. Pour the boiling water into the jar over the plant material; try to leave as little air as possible. Screw the lid on tightly. Let it steep at room temperature:
- For flowers: two hours
- For leaves: four to six hours
- For flowers and leaves: four hours
- For seeds and berries: 30 minutes
- For roots and bark: eight hours or overnight
- Strain the infusion when it is ready.

REGULAR DECOCTION FOR MOST ROOTS AND BARKS:

INGREDIENTS:

1 ounce (medium handful) of dried root or bark, 2 cups of cold water

1. Cover and simmer (slowly) for twenty minutes. Do not boil. Strain. Can be kept in the fridge for two to three days.

2. Roots and bark can be soaked in the same amount of water overnight before simmering; this increases their potency.
   Berries and Seeds
1. Grind lightly.
2. Use 3 teaspoons for every 3 cups of water.
3. Cover and simmer for twenty minutes. Do not boil. Strain and drink three cups a day.

NORMAL DOSAGE (ADULTS)

infusions 1/4 to 1 cup, three to four times a day (unless specified otherwise); dosages for each individual plant are specified in the chapter, "Herbal Properties and Dosages". Take for a period of six to twelve weeks depending on the change desired. Hormones take a little longer to persuade to change.

DECOCTIONS

Take two ounces (1/4 cup) three to four times a day, unless specified otherwise. Dosages for each individual plant are specified in the chapter, "Herbal Properties and Dosages".

It is recommended to take the herb six days a week for a period of six weeks. This process can be repeated several times, unless specified otherwise. We have to keep in mind that everyone's body reacts differently to herbs (according to weight, age, etc...). To adapt our needs, we can slightly increase or decrease the quantities and duration of the treatments. Use your best judgement.

TINCTURES

This contains the alkaloid parts of the plant, extracted and preserved in alcohol. As they are concentrated herbal extracts, they maintain their potency, are easy to prepare, act quickly , can be carried, and ingested easily. They are sold in herb stores and health food stores. While tinctures may seem expensive (their prices range from $9 to $14 per dropper bottle), they last a very long time. Consider the fact that antibiotics can cost anywhere from $20 to $60 a bottle, for a seven day dose!

Tinctures are used diluted in warm water (about 30 drops in a little bit of water, three times a day). Surprisingly, they are easy to make.

TO MAKE YOUR OWN TINCTURES:

- Always use fresh plant material: flowers, stems, and leaves. Dried plant can work for some tinctures. Everclear alcohol or 45 percent vodka is usually best.
- Dried roots can be used but are not as potent as fresh ones.
- Brown glass bottles with droppers can be bought in some health food stores. These are used to measure the dosage. Use only glass droppers as plastic ones can be easily contaminated.
- Useful tinctures to keep on hand are: valerian, echinacea, and yarrow.
- Use a clean, dry mason jar with a tight-fitting lid. It's not a bad idea to boil it first, to make sure it's sterile (let it dry out completely before starting your tincture).

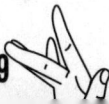

- Do not wash or rinse plant material. Fresh roots can be scrubbed or peeled.
- Coarsely chop the parts of the plant you are using (with the exception of small flowers). Fill jar to the top with fresh herbs and add vodka or Everclear to the rim.
- If using dried herbs, fill jar one-fifth of the way and then add vodka. If using grain alcohol, fill half way and the rest with distilled water.
- Use a knife to dislodge any air bubbles. Make sure to fill the jar to the top and cap it as tightly as possible. Label the jar with the name of the plant used and the date. Make one tincture for each plant you are using.
- One of the most important aspects of making a tincture is the daily agitation of it. This is necessary as it is the shaking that helps further the break down of plant material allowing the healing constituents to be drawn from it into the liquid. Therefore, be sure to shake it vigorously each and every day. Set it somewhere where you'll be sure to remember.
- The tincture will be ready in six weeks. When it's ready, strain, squeeze, and discard the plant matter.
- Store your tinctures in sterilized brown glass bottles, away from light and in a cool place.

CAPSULES

These use ground or powdered herbs (ex. cayenne pepper, ginger). You can buy empty vegetable capsules (size 00 to be precise) at health food or herb stores and fill them up yourself. This is cheaper than buying ready-made ones.

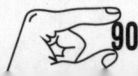

POULTIC

This is essentially crushed plant material, applied externally to the infected area (sores, cuts, burns, etc.). For fresh plants, chop or grate the plant material and apply it directly to the affected area; it is okay for application on open wounds.

- Pour boiling water over the plant, cover and soak for half an hour to four hours.
- Strain, squeeze the water out and apply them to the affected areas. Make sure temperature is cool enough, to avoid burning the affected area.
- You can also wrap poultices in a thin layer of gauze before applying. The liquid can be used as an infusion or a soak.

WASH (ALSO KNOWN AS A SOAK)

This is an infusion which is reheated, never boiled, and then applied externally to the affected areas. Soak the area directly in the wash, or dip a clean cloth into the wash and apply it wherever needed.

PASTE

A paste is made by mixing the powdered herb with a small amount of water, then applied externally to the affected area.

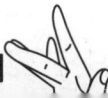

Douches can cause as much damage as they resolve. Force can worsen an infection by sending it up into your uterus, which can then cause PID. Instead, gently wash the genitals, which can be quite effective.

SYRINGES

"Baby syringes" are relatively large syringes (about an inch in diameter) with an opening at the tip. They do not have a needle. They can be found in many pharmacies. There are also plastic vaginal medicine applicators that come with certain products, such as Vagisil, which are designed to safely deliver the medicine up the vagine.

Certain infusions and decoctions do not taste very good. You can add honey and lemon. Most preparations should be taken warm unless specified otherwise. For long-term treatments, remember that tinctures are another option.

Most of the plants used and mentioned in this book grow in North America and are therefore available in both the city and the country, as well as many herb/health stores. Keep in mind that herbs are not drugs but foods. They provide nourishment for the body to heal itself. Although some herbs are not to be taken during pregnancy, there are generally no side effects. It is a normal reaction, however, to have less of an appetite and/or light diarrhea during a treatment. You may have to urinate often. Always drink lots of water during a treatment, as it is important to stay hydrated in order to flush the herbs out and avoid damage to the liver and kidneys.

Don't hesitate to seek help from experts in your area and remember that certain chronic problems or acute conditions will need more individualized treatment.

PICKING YOUR OWN HERBS

Several of the plants mentioned in this book are easily found growing in the countryside; many of them are also commonly found in gardens and empty lots in the city. Chamomile (page 101), chickweed (page 101), red raspberry leaves (page 111), tansy (page 114), wild carrot seed (page 117) and yarrow (page 118) are among the most abundant and easiest to spot.

Picking your own herbs gives you the advantage of getting the freshest herbs possible, allowing you to prepare your own tinctures and dried herbs, and it can also save you money.

However, if you do want to pick your own herbs, there are a few things you should know.

1. Some plants are poisonous and even deadly if ingested; for example, wild carrot seed is easily confused with poison hemlock, which can be fatal). You should be 100 percent sure that the plant you are picking is really the

one you want! Unless you've done this before, it's best to go on a "field trip" with someone who knows their stuff, in addition to consulting a field-guide book to help you recognize and identify plants. Familiarize yourself with the plants; take note of how they look and smell before you embark on picking anything. If you're ever unsure, don't take chances. Always take a field-guide book with you.

2. Be respectful. Never pick more than a third of the plants available. This ensures they will come back the following year.

3. It's far better to pick plants in the country rather than in the city. If you must pick them in the city, get them from parks or empty lots located far from roads—otherwise you may be wasting your time. Plants located near roadways are high in lead and other toxic, chemical contaminants.

4. Read up on the subject. Know when to pick the plants and plant parts you need. For example, roots are best harvested in the fall, flowers right after they bloom, etc.

FOR FURTHER READING

The Wise Women Herbal: Healing Wise
by Susun S. Weed

Peterson Field Guides to Medicinal Plants (Houghton Mifflin
Company) are excellent for identifying plants. The one we
use here in Ontario and Quebec is the Eastern/Central
Guide. Other guides in North America and even Central
and South America are also available.

A City Herbal by Maida Silverman. 1977. Knopf.

*The Chinese Medicine Bible: The Definitive Guide to Holistic
Healing* by Penelope Ody. 2011. Sterling

*Reclaiming Our Ancient Wisdom: Herbal Abortion Procedure
and Practice for Midwives and Herbalists* by Catherine Marie
Jeunet. 2007. Eberhardt Press.

*Born in the USA: How a Broken Maternity System Must Be
Fixed to Put Women and Children First* by Marsden Wagner.
2008. Univ of Cal

Witches, Midwives, and Nurses: A History of Women Healers by
Barbara Ehrenreich. 2010. Feminist Press

The Herbal Apothecary: 100 Herbs to Know and Use by Dr. JJ
Pursell. 2015. Timber Press

HERBAL PROPERTIES AND DOSAGES

The English and French common names (eg. bearberry in English; busserole in French) of the plants are provided, as are their Latin names (eg. Arctostaphylos ova ours). When buying herbs, always take note of the Latin name of the plant you need; this will ensure that you get exactly what you're looking for. It's also helpful for buying herbs in non-English or French speaking regions or countries.

Consuming caffeine, nicotine, alcohol, and sugar interferes with the absorption of plant material, vitamins and minerals, making the treatments less effective. Try to limit your intake of these substances when using herbal remedies.

If you buy herbs, make sure you buy good quality, well-preserved dried herbs. Dried herbs remain potent for about twelve months. Store them in brown paper bags or glass jars in a cool, dark place. Commercially sold herbs should be colorful and aromatic. Buy herbs that have not been sprayed with pesticides or other chemicals. Consult the resources section for a list of reliable herb stores and mail-order distributors.

When we talk about using the whole plant, we mean the stems, leaves and flowers: this does not include the plant's root.

Bearberry (Uva-Ursi)
Arctostaphylos uva-ursi/ busserole
part used: leaves

Bearberry acts specifically on the genital—urinary system. Acting as a diuretic, we use it to treat the prostate, cystitis, the kidneys, bladder inflammation, uterine and vaginal infections.

An active ingredient in bearberry is a toxic chemical known as hydroquinone; nausea or dizziness are common side effects. Long- term use without qualified supervision is not recommended.

Infusion: To make a regular infusion (page 73), take 1/2 cup, three to four times daily.

Blue Cohosh Root
Caulophyllum thalictroides/ act blue
part used: root

Blue cohosh is used to treat amenorrhea, dysmenorrhea, vaginal inflammation, suppressed and cramping periods, slow or halted contractions (during childbirth), nervousness, exhaustion and spasmodic cough (asthma, bronchitis, whooping cough).

Do not use during pregnancy, or in cases of high blood pressure or heart disease. The seeds of this plant are poisonous.

Make a regular decoction (page 73). Take 1 teaspoon-1 tablespoon, three to four times a day.

For amenorrhea and dysmenorrhea: 1/4 cup of the hot decoction, three times a day.

Spasms: Take stronger doses or ingest more often.

Cayenne Pepper
Capiscum frutescens/ poivre de cayenne
part used: fruit

Cayenne pepper (also known as cayenne powder, as it most often comes in powdered form) is a stimulant, tonic, astringent, blood-cleanser, and antiseptic. It induces sweating and is excellent for blood circulation, stimulating the heart, regulating blood pressure, relieving congestion in the mucus membrane, and cleaning and restoring elasticity to the veins and arteries, allowing excessive blood flow in the lining of the uterus to be decreased. It can help soothe and heal sores in the stomach and intestinal tissues, as well as accelerate coagulation and stop both internal and external bleeding. Cayenne is effective in cases of anorexia and liver congestion, and is a great source of physical energy. It also strengthens the immune system and is excellent for colds and asthma. Be sure to buy only medicinal cayenne pepper. It is also sold as a kitchen spice, but in this form it is roasted and devoid of its therapeutic properties. Consult your local herb store.

For colds: 1/4 to 1 teaspoon in very hot water, three times daily.

Capsules: 1/4 to 1 teaspoon in a capsule taken with a hot beverage, three times per day.

Celery Seed
Apium graveolens/ graines de celeri
part used: seed

Celery seed is a diuretic. It will lower high blood pressure, as well as relieve headaches and anxiety. The seeds are high in flavonoids, antioxidants, volatile oils, and linoleic acid.

Infusion: Grind lightly and put 3 teaspoons in 3 cups of cold water. Cover and simmer for 20 minutes. Strain. Drink hot, three cups daily.

Chamomile

Matricaria chamomilla or
Matricaria recutita/ camomille
part used: flowers

Chamomile is a sedative for the nerves and a tonic for the intestines. It is used for earaches, toothaches, for slow or difficult digestion, insomnia and the flu. For those who are pollen sensitvie, take caution of this herb's flowers.

Infusion: 1/2 ounce of flowers, in 3 cups of water. Take 1/2 to one cup, three to four times in a day.

For colds: 1/4 teaspoon of cayenne powder in 1 cup of chamomile infusion; add honey. Drink hot, four to five times a day.

Chickweed

Stellaria media/ ceraiste vulgaire
part used: whole plant

Chickweed can grow in both city and country settings; it is best to collect when young and bright green. It is an expectorant, a laxative, relieves gas and colic, helps soothe and protect mucus membranes, and promotes healing both externally and internally. Fresh chickweed can dissolve warts; in tincture form it is effective in dissolving cysts, especially ovarian cysts. The leaves can be made into a poultice (page 75) or wash (page 76) to treat external infections and irritations, including pinkeye. Be aware- chickweed has a look-alike that often grows in close quarter with it, scarlet pimpernel. This can cause constipation, inflammation, head pains, nausea and kidney problems.

Infusion: Make a regular infusion. Drink 1/2 cup, three to four times a day.

For constipation: Take one cup of the infusion every three hours.

Tincture: 15 to 20 drops in a glass of warm water, two to three times a day. (This can be used as a long-term treatment for cysts.)

Fresh plant: The more you eat, the better!

Cinnamon
Cinnamomum zeylanicum/ cannelle
part used: bark

Cinnamon is useful in case of muscular pains, flu, and digestive spasms. It is also an aphrodisiac.

Decoction: Make a normal decoction: take one-fourth of a cup three to four times daily.

Cloves
Eugenia caryophyllata/ clou de girofle
part used: dried flowers and buds

Cloves facilitate circulation, raise body temperature, stimulate and disinfect the stomach, skin, kidneys, intestines, lungs, and bronchi. Clove oil is an analgesic that stops toothaches when applied directly to the tooth or cavity.

Infusion: 1 teaspoon of cloves in 2 cups water. Take one-eighth of a cup three times daily.

Echinacea (Purple Coneflower)
Echinacea pupurea or augustifolia/ rudbeckie
part used: root

A blood purifier, it stimulates the production of white blood cells which destroy bacteria and viruses. Echinacea is an herbal substitute for antibiotics as it strengthens the immune system in times of need. It is also used for blood poisoning, poisonous stings and bites, chronic or acute bacterial infections, vaginal infections (such as yeast infections), and hemorrhoids. A good prostate tonic, it can facilitate the elimination of fat. Echinacea is non-toxic but should not be taken over long periods of time.

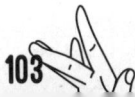

Decoction: Make a regular decoction. Add licorice root if the taste makes you feel nauseous. Take 1 to 5 tablespoons, three to six times a day.

Tincture: Fifteen to thirty drops in a little warm water every one to six hours, depending on the gravity of the infection.

Garlic
Allium satvium/ ail
part used: bulb

Raw garlic is a natural antiseptic and blood purifier. It regulates circulation, as well as blood pressure, and can also help treat yeast infections, chlamydia, and nervous disorders. It is a diuretic, helps balance glandular disorders, and strengthens the immune system. It is also an estrogenic, and can be used as a suppository.

It's also good for warts, earaches, and corns.

For all treatments, we recommend organic or homegrown garlic.

Raw garlic: Chop or press garlic clove. Take with cold water or mix with honey. Don't wait more than five minutes after you cut the clove to consume it. Eat one or more cloves of fresh garlic three to four times a day.

Earache (ear infection): Peel one garlic clove without breaking it. Wrap it in cheesecloth or gauze. Dip it in olive oil and put in the opening of the ear (DON'T push it too far in) before going to bed, and if possible, during the day, for four days or more. Also eat fresh garlic.

Warts: Rub the wart with a garlic clove cut in half as often as possible. Keep in mind this may burn.

Ginger
Zingiber officinale/ gingembre
part used: rhizome and root

Ginger is a stimulant, an analgesic, and an aphrodisiac. It is used for boils, bronchitis, colic pain, diarrhea, the flu, sore throats, hemorrhage of the lungs, painful menstruation, nausea, neuralgia, rheumatism, and is particularly effective for abdominal problems. It can also help bring on a late period. It can be taken in capsules with a hot beverage or be added to your bath for fever and skin irritations. It can be used as a powder, but the fresh root of an organic plant is the most potent form. Consuming large doses of ginger may result in nausea.

Infusion: Fresh ginger: Grate a good quantity of the root and infuse in boiled water for 30 to 60 minutes.

Powdered ginger: 1 teaspoon per cup of hot water with honey and lemon. Drink one cup three times a day with honey. For

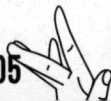

colds, add 1/4 teaspoon cayenne pepper to each cup.

Capsules: Fill capsules with ginger powder, take three capsules daily.

Fresh root: Simply chew a good quantity of the root several times a day with water, or grate it and mix with honey.

Golden Seal Root
Hyrastis canadensis/ hydraste canadien
part used: root and rhizome

Similar to echinacea and myrrh, goldenseal root is a powerful natural antibiotic used for viral and bacterial infections. Goldenseal is a remedy for severe inflammations of the nose, throat, stomach, colon, and also good for hemorrhoids, ulcers, acne, ringworm, dandruff or herpes-type viruses (cold sores, shingles). It is an excellent eyewash for conjunctivitis, antiseptic mouthwash for infected gums and sore throats, wash for yeast infections or as treatment for skin problems or burns. Keep in mind, it will temporarily stain the skin yellow.

Infusion: 1/4 teaspoon of powdered root in 1 cup boiling water. Mix well. Take 2 to 5 tablespoons four times a day.

Capsules: Measure 1/4 tablespoon of powder. Fill three capsules with this amount. Take three capsules daily.

Tincture: Fifteen drops in warm water three times a day.

Paste: Mix small amount of powder with water to make a

light paste. Use externally on skin infections and cover with a cloth, as it stains.

WARNING: Goldenseal is toxic when used excessively. Do not use for longer than two weeks. Do not use during pregnancy or when breastfeeding. People with high blood pressure or problems with their liver or heart should first consult an herb practitioner before taking.

Lavender
Lavendula officinalis/ lavande
part used: flowers

Lavender is a sedative and an antibacterial. Use the essential oil externally on open sores, to soothe insect bites, and also to treat yeast infections. Wash it off after about fifteen to twenty minutes, as it can burn. For a relaxing bath, prepare an infusion off fresh, organic lavender and add to the water or add a few drops of lavender essential oil. Be cautious of headaches or nausea that may follow after topical treatment or inhaling of lavender. It should only be taken internally under supervision.

Licorice
Glycyrrhiza glabara/ reglisse
**Part used: the whole root, broken into pieces
or in powder form**

Licorice is an emollient, an expectorant, and a gentle laxative. It is used in the treatment of colds, ulcers, colic, sore throats, heartburn, and it exhibits anti-inflammatory effects. It also contains substances similar to estrogen (as does sage). In Chinese medicine its nickname is "the reconcilor" since in addition to being used on its own, it can be combined with all other herbs. Its presence increases their medicinal properties while masking the bitter taste of some herbs. We do warn against licorice in some cases, as it has caused trouble for people with PVCs from hypokalemia; especially people with kidney problems or diabetes. Do not take if you have high blood pressure, kidney issues or are pregnant. It is also highly estrogenic; use with caution and know how much you are consuming.

Decoction: 1 ounce or more of licorice root. Simmer for twenty minutes in 2 cups of water. Take 1/4 cup three to four times a day. This quantity can be added to other decoctions or infusions.

Laxative: 1 teaspoon of powder mixed with honey. Chewing on the dried root (in stick form) helps regulate digestive problems as well.

Motherwort
Leonorus cardiaca/ agripaume
part used: leaves

A really good uterine and heart tonic, motherwort also relieves cramps. It is ideal for regulating menstruation, or temporarily relieving the anxiety and heart-palpitations, which may follow childbirth or menopause. It can be used in strong doses and for long periods of time. Do not use during pregnancy.

Infusion: Make a regular infusion. Drink 1/4th cup three to four times a day.

Late menstruation: Drink warm. When the flow is normal, drink cold as a tonic.

Mugwort
Artemisia vulgaris/ armoise
part used: whole plant

Emmenagogue, anti-epileptic, anti-spasmodic. Can also activate one's digestive system as well as stimulate the liver. Contains thujone, do not takr for longer than two weeks, in case of uterine inflammation or during pregnancy. It is also not advised for mothers who are nursing, as it may dry up the milk.

Make a regular infusion. Take 1/4th cup three to four

times a day.

Parsley
Petroselinum satvium/ persil
part used: whole plant

Parsley is rich in minerals and contains more iron than any other green vegetable. It is rich in vitamin A and B and has three times more vitamin C than citrus fruits. Parsley is excellent for kidneys and bladder stones, also good for the suprarenal glands, blood vessels, and both optical and cervical nerves. It prevents rheumatism, helps inflamed glands, and prevents menstrual problems. It increases a mother's breast milk and strengthens the uterine muscles. The roots and seeds are used in decoction. If you have a hard time eating enough fresh parsley, take it in infusion instead. In case of kidney infection, take ginger (which is anti-inflammatory) instead. Keep in mind organic or homegrown parsley is best. Avoid medicinal use when pregnant.

Infusion: Make a regular infusion. Take two to six tablespoons four times a day.

Red Raspberry Leaves
rubus idaeus/ feuilles de framboisier
part used: leaves

Red raspberry leaves are used for diarrhea, hemorrhoids, vaginitis, hormonal problems, and during and after pregnancy. They are by far one of the best uterine tonics. They stimulate menstrual flow by toning the ovaries and uterus and improving their functions. Taken during menstruation, red raspberry leaves relieve cramps and regulate the flow. They also help with digestion and nausea. Taken during pregnancy, it can strengthen the mother's immune system, as well as tone pelvic muscles to better prepare for childbirth. Be cautious in your use of this herb, it is believed to be estrogenic and may exacerbate uterine and cervical cancers and endometriosis.

This herb also contains a high level of tannins. Due to the astringent properties of tannins, they can help with diarrhea and have anti-inflammatory properties, but can impair absorptions of calcium, iron, Mg and certain prescriptions.

Infusion: Make a regular infusion. Take 1 cup three times daily.

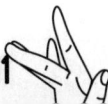

Rosehips
Rosa canina/ eglantier
part used: fruit

A tonic for fatigue and vitamin deficiencies and a diuretic, rosehips contain a lot of vitamin C. They are excellent for the skin and help balance hormonal irregularities, also good for irregular menstrual cycles and heavy white vaginal discharge (leucorrhea leukorrhea). They also work as a mild laxative.

Make a regular infusion. Take the recommended dosage (page 63). Rosehips in infusion are excellent cold with lemon.

Rosemary
Rosemarinus officinalis/ romarin
part used: leaves

Often used for headaches, poor circulation, colic pains, colds, nervousness, depression, palpitations and uterine congestion. A pulmonary cleanser, it is also helpful for asthma when the steam is inhaled. It can help in treating painful periods and strengthening blood vessels. Add a strong infusion to your bath. Or take an infusion or apply directly to head for headaches. Undiluted oil should not be internally consumed.

Make a regular infusion; drink 1/4 cup, three to four times a day.

Sage
Salvia officinalis/ sauge
part used: leaves

Used for sore throats, mouth ulcers, bringing down high fevers, painful periods and for stimulating circulation and digestion. This herb imitates estrogen and can help with certain menstrual irregularities as well as impairing lactation. It also has oestrogenic properties, rendering it useful in cases of hot flashes brought on by menopause. Use fresh, organic sage. In the case of sage tea, only take for one to two weeks at a time due to it's toxic ingredient and FDA controlled substance, Thujone.

Infusion: Make a regular infusion. Take one to three times a day.

To impair lactation: one cup of cold infusion twice a day.

To gargle with: Make an infusion using 1/2 cup of water and 1/2 cup of apple cider vinegar.

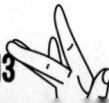

Tansy (Bitter Buttons)
Tanacetum vulgare/ tanaisie vulgaire
part used: leaves, flowers and seeds

Tansy is used for amenorrhea and dysmenorrhea. The seeds can be used to expel worms. It is an emmenagogue which can be used to promote regular periods. Take in small, repeated doses. Extra large doses can cause congestion and result in discomfort to the abdominal organs. Like sage, it contains Thujone, and thus can be quite toxic if taken in large quantities. Externally, tansy tea is used for the treatment of scabies and to relieve rheumatic joints.

Warning: Tansy can cause heavy bleeding in women who usually have a heavy flow. It is phototoxic, and may also cause temporary lumps in the breast of females who use it for the purpose of menstruation. Do not confuse with Tansy Ragwort.

Infusion: Prepare a regular infusion using 1 ounce Tansy to 1 pint (500 ml) water. Take one cup three times a day before meals.

Tincture: Ten to fifteen drops in warm water, three to four times a day.

Thyme

Thymus vulgaris or Thymus pulegeoides/ thym
part used: leaves

Thyme is an antibacterial and antifungal. It is used for headaches, fever, colds, bronchitis, cramps, digestive problems, nightmares, whooping cough, wounds, toothaches, scabies, sore throats, ulcers, worms, rheumatism, and also as a deodorant or mouthwash. Thyme tea can be useful in treatment of yeast infections. Organic or homegrown thyme is best.

Infusion: 1 teaspoon of thyme in 1 cup of water. Drink one cup, three to four times a day.

For cough: Mix with honey; take 1 to 2 teaspoons as needed.

For fever: Drink as a hot infusion. Wrap yourself in blankets so as to sweat; then shower.

For worms: One to five drops of thyme essential oil with honey and some olive oil, three times daily.

For skin problems, scabies, and parasites: Mix 2 to 3 teaspoons of thyme essential oil in 5 ounces of olive oil. Apply three or more times a day to the affected areas. Take thyme infusions three times a day as well.

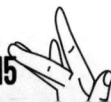

Valerian
Valeriana officinalis/ valeriane
part used: root

Valerian is used in cases of anxiety, depression, digestion or circulation disorders. It is good for treating anxiety, spasms, trembling, convulsions, heart palpitations, epilepsy, and neuralgia and can also remedy problems with sleeping, headaches, and pain in general. It also helps to relieve menstrual cramps. Only take valerian if advised by an herbal practitioner—it may cause palpitations, muscle spasms, and headaches. Avoid prolonged use.

Prepare valerian as an infusion only, never as a decoction. Do not presoak the roots or steep longer than two hours.

Due to its bitter taste and foul smell, it is suggested to add one of the following medicinal herbs to valerian infusions: cinnamon (for convulsions), cayenne (for cramps), anise (for digestive disorders), ginger (for menstrual irregularities).

Infusion: 1 ounce of the root. 2 cups of boiling water. Steep covered for 45 minutes. Take 1/4th of a cup three to four times a day.

Tincture: Ten to fifteen drops in a little water, three to four times a day.

Wild Carrot Seed
(Queen Anne's Lace)
Daueus carota/ carotte sauvage
part used: seeds, roots

Root tea is a diuretic which helps eliminate urinary stones and worms.

The seeds are rich in volatile oil and can be used as a "morning after pill" to prevent the implantation of a fertilized egg, particularly if the egg has only been implanted for a short time (see page 32). It can also be used to bring on menstruation. Its pulpy root is ideal as a poultice for itchy skin. It can grow in both the city and countryside, thriving along the roads or in fields. Keep in mind it is also an estrogenic.

Warning: Be very careful about identifying this plant. It is easily confused with poison hemlock, which can cause death.

Yarrow
Achillea millefolium/ achillee mille-feuille
part used: flowers and leaves

Yarrow is a cleanser and an anti-inflammatory. It is used for colds and the flu, hemorrhages of the lungs and the intestines, vaginal and bladder infections, menstrual disorders, hemorrhoids, headaches, fatigue, and circulation problems. It acts to lower blood pressure by encouraging blood flow to the skin, and can also treat both external and internal bleeding. In tincture form, it can help alleviate cramps and problems with hormones. It is not to be taken during pregnancy. It may also increase one's sensitivity to sunlight.

Infusions: Make a regular infusion. Drink three to four cups daily.

Decoction: Start with a regular infusion that's been prepared and strained. Simmer until the liquid is reduced to half of its original volume. Strain and drink cold; half a cup, three times a day.

For flu and colds: Drink one to two cups of the hot infusion. For colds, wrap yourself in blankets after drinking in order to sweat, then take a bath.

For abdominal pain/heavy bleeding: Take a hot infusion before menstruation or as needed for cramps.

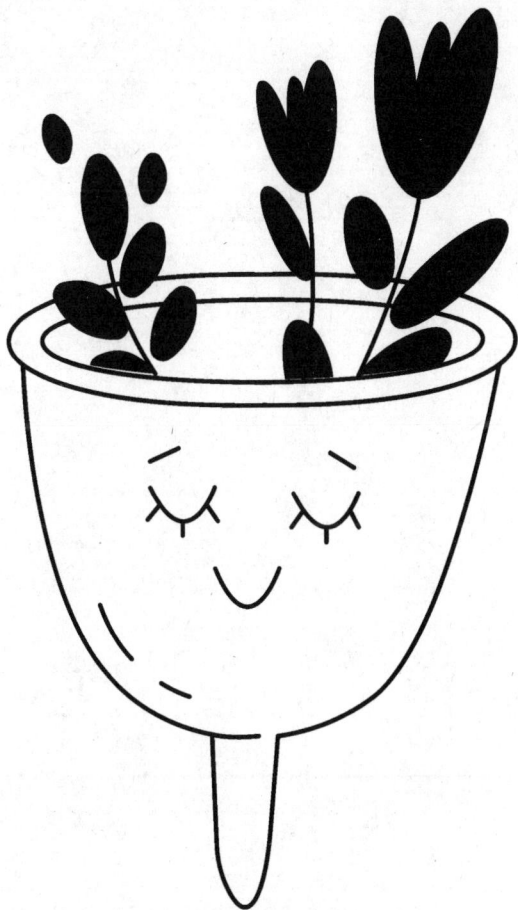

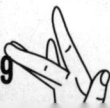

GLOSSARY

AIDS—acquired immune deficiency syndrome, a disease in which there is a severe loss of the body's cellular immunity, greatly lowering the resistance to infection and malignancy.

anus—the opening at the end of the alimentary canal through which solid waste matter leaves the body.

aphrodisiacs—an herb that stimulates sexual desire

aromatic essences—see essential oils

baby syringe—large syringe with an opening at the top which are used to insert things into the vagina

bacterial infections—the growth of many infection-causing bacteria

Bartholin's abscess (or cyst)—formed when a Bartholin's gland is blocked, causing a fluid-filled cyst to develop. A Bartholin's cyst is not an infection, although it can be caused by an infection, inflammation, or physical blockage to the Bartholin's ducts.

Bartholin's glands—located at the opening of the vestibule and secrete fluid during stimulation

bladder infection—see urinary infection

candida—a yeastlike, parasitic fungus

capsule—ground or powdered solution

cervical canal—the source of cervical mucus

cervix—the narrow necklike passage forming the lower end of the uterus

chlamydia—a very small parasitic bacterium that, like a virus, requires the biochemical mechanisms of another cell in order to reproduce.

clitoris—an external female genital organ

contraception—a deliberate method to prevent pregnancy as a consequence of sexual intercourse

crabs—a louse that infests human body hair, especially in the genital region, that causes extreme irritation

decoction—the liquor resulting from concentrating the essence of a substance by heating or boiling a medicinal preparation made from a plant

dental dams—triangular rubber sheaths used for performing safe sex

discharge—vaginal mucus

Don Quai—Traditionally a Chinese herb, it is known for its ability to ease cramps and other symptoms of PMS, balance estrogen levels, induce relaxation, encourage a more regular cycle, promote a more healthy blood flow during a woman's menstruation, and is an excellent blood toner. Women who have uterine fibroids or who are pregnant or nursing are not advised to take up treatment.

emmenagogues—herbs which encourage menstrual flow by promoting uterine contractions

endometrium—the mucous membrane lining the uterus, which thickens during the menstrual cycle in preparation for possible implantation of an embryo.

essential oils—a natural oil obtained by distilling a plant or other herb

estrogen—any of a group of steroid hormones that promise the development and maintenance of female characteristics of the body

fallopian tubes—connected to the uterus, which harbors the ovum

fibroid—a fiber or fibrous tissue

gardnarella—genus of Gram-variable-staining facultative anaerobic bacteria of which G. vaginalis is the only species

genital warts (venereal warts)—small growths occurring in the anal or genital areas, caused by a virus that is spread especially by sexual contact.

GLOSSARY

gonorrhea—a veneral disease involving inflammatory discharge from the urethra or vagina

gynecologist—a doctor specializing in the physciology and medicine of those specific to the female reproductive system

gynecology—the branch of physiology and medicine that deals with the functions and diseases specific to women and girls, esp. those affecting the reproductive system.

herpes simplex 1— an infection of the lips, mouth, or gums due to the herpes simplex virus. It causes small, painful blisters commonly called cold sores or fever blisters.

herpes simplex 11—a virus that causes genital herpes, which is characterized by sores in the genital area.

HIV—(human immunodeficiency virus) a retrovirus that causes AIDS.

hymen-a membrane that partially closes the opening of the vagina and whose presence is traditionally taken to be a mark of virginity.

hypothalamus—a region of the forebrain below the thalamus that coordinates both the autonomic nervous system and the activity of the pituitary, controlling body temperature, thirst, hunger, and other homeostatic systems, and involved in sleep and emotional activity.

infertility—the inability to reproduce

infusion—a drink, remedy, or extract prepared by soaking the leaves of a plant or herb in liquid.

labia—an external female genital organ

labia majora—outer lips that cover the vulva

labia minora—inside the labia majora

menstrual cycle—the process of ovulation and menstruation in women

menstruation—the process in a woman of discharging blood and other materials from the lining of the uterus at intervals of about one lunar month from puberty until menopause, except during pregnancy.

myectomy—removal of the fibrous tumor

ovaries—a female reproductive organ in which ova or eggs are produced, present in humans and other vertebrates as a pair.

ovarian cysts—a sac filled with fluid that forms on or inside of an ovary.

ovulation—discharge ova or ovules from the ovary.

ovum—multiple ova or eggs

pap smear—a test to detect cancer of the cervix or uterus, using a specimen of cellular material from the neck of the uterus spread on a microscope slide

paste—a mixture of a powdered herb and small amount of water which is then applied to an affected area

pelvic inflammatory disease—inflammation of the female genital tract, accompanied by fever and lower abdominal pain.

Peppermint—A well-known ingredient in many teas and foods, peppermint is also used to treat sinus and respiratory problems, nausea, morning sickness, vomiting, and menstrual problems.

perineum—the muscle between the anus and vagina

The Pill—a pill taken to avoid pregnancy

pituitary gland—a pea-sized body attached to the base of the brain, the pituitary is important in controlling growth and development and the functioning of the other endocrine glands. also called hypophysis and is the major endocrine gland.

poultice—essential crushed plant material applied externally to the

GLOSSARY

infected area

progesterone—a steroid hormone released by the corpus luteum that stimulates the uterus to prepare for pregnancy.

prostaglandins-a group of cyclic fatty acid compounds with varying hormonelike effects, notably the promotion of uterine contractions.

safe sex—sexual activity in which people take precautions to protect themselves against sexually transmitted diseases and infections

scabies—a contagious skin disease marked by itching and small raised red spots, caused by the itch mite.

Sheperd's purse—Named after the sack-like shape of its seeds, it can be used to treat both internal and external bleeding, as well as urinary infections, menorrhagia, and varicose veins. A uterine stimulant, it is also useful in aiding with urinary contractions. Not recommended for long term consumption.

sitz bath—a bath in which only the buttocks and hips are immersed in water.

Skene's glands—attached to the vulva, under the clitoris

speculum—a metal or plastic instrument that is used to dilate an orifice or canal in the body to allow inspection.

STD—sexually transmitted disease.

STI-sexually transmitted infection

tinctures—contain the alkaloid part of a plant, extracted and preserved in alcohol

toxic shock syndrome-acute septicemia in women, typically caused by bacterial infection from a retained tampon or IUD.

trichomonas—a sexually transmitted infection caused by the parasite

Trichomonas vaginalis.

urethra-the duct by which urine is conveyed out of the body from the bladder, and which in male vertebrates also conveys semen.

urinary infection—an infection that can happen anywhere along the urinary tract

vagina—the channel which connects the vulva and internal organs

vaginitis—inflammation of the vagina.

vestibule—the space between the labia minora

venereal disease—see std

venereal infection—see sti

vulvitis—inflammation of the vulva.

wash—an infusion that is reheated then applied externally to the affected area

yeast infection—infection of the vagina with an overgrowth of a normally present candidal fungus that is characterized by a discharge and inflammation

We hope this book will inspire you to
seek out more alternative information and
explore your options.

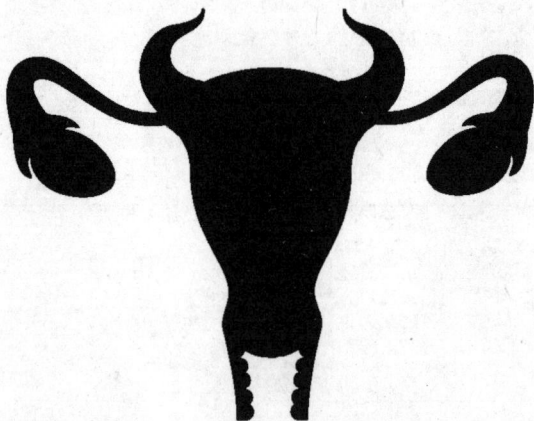

AT YOUR
CERVIX!

ACKNOWLEDGEMENTS

Special thanks for inspiration to Joyce Rediker, La Fee des Roses, Susun Weed, Sue Ann Harkey.

Women are encouraged to share this information amongst themselves. You can download a photocopyable version here: www.indybay.org/uploads/2010/04/06/hotpantz.pdf

Microcosm donated 400 copies of this work to shelters and clinics for at-risk women. Donations sent for this purpose can help us expand this outreach.

ABOUT THE AUTHORS

Isabelle Gauthier holds a degree in herbal therapy. She studied with Joyce Rediker of Le Grand Monde des Herbes in Montreal, and has been an herbal practitioner since 1991.

Lisa Vinebaum is a community radio activist. She has been using herbal therapy on herself and selected patients for a number of years.

What started as a way to restore her own body evolved into a journey of education and experience to bring healing to others. This passion led **JJ Pursell** to receive a Doctorate in Naturopathic Medicine and Acupuncture in Portland, OR— learning to bring balance to body and soul through western and alternative medicine practices. She is an author, speaker, researcher, entrepreneur, and healer.

Jennifer Baumgardner has been working in NYC publishing since her 1993 unpaid internship at *Ms.* She led the Feminist Press and *Women's Review of Books*. Jennifer now runs Dottir Press, which publishes books for all ages and is writer-in-residence at Smith College.

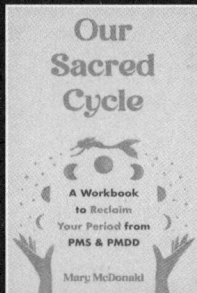

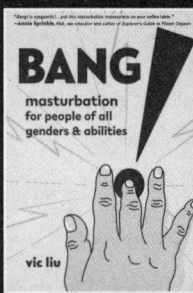

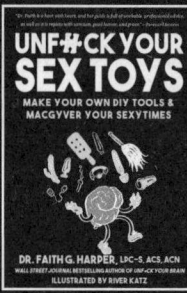

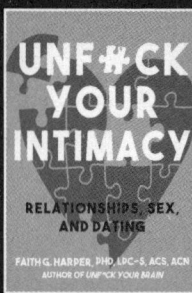

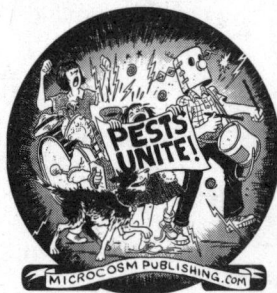

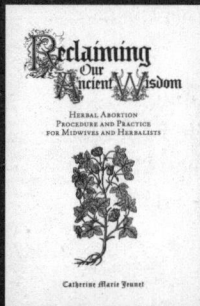

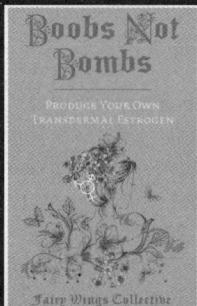

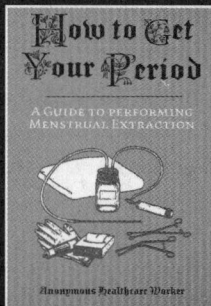

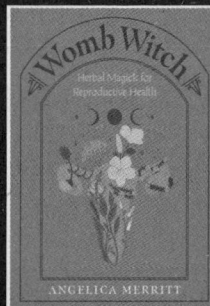